PAIN MANAGEMENT

for

CHRONIC BACK PAIN SUFFERERS

PROF. GEORGE ZAFIROPOULOS

Copyright @George Zafiropoulos

ALL RIGHTS RESERVED: No part of this book may be reproduced or transmitted in any form whatsoever, electronic, or mechanical, including photocopying, recording, or by any informational storage or retrieval system without the express written, dated, and signed permission from the author.

Author: George Zafiropoulos @2024
Title: Pain Management For Chronic Back Pain Sufferers

ISBN: 978-1-7384171-6-2
Category: Personal Development/Self-help/Health

Publisher: Breakfree Forever Publishing

LIMITS OF LIABILITY/DISCLAIMER OF WARRANTY: The author and publisher of this book has used their best efforts in preparing this material. The author and publisher make no representation or warranties with respect to the accuracy, applicability, or completeness of the contents. They disclaim any warranties (expressed or implied), or merchantability for any particular purpose. The author andpublisher shall in no event be held liable for any loss or other damages, including but not limited to special, incidental, consequential, or other damages. The information presented in this publication is compiled from sources believed to be accurate. However, the publisher assumes no responsibility forerrors or omissions. The information in this publication is not intended to replace or substituteprofessional advice. The author and publisher specifically disclaim any liability, loss, or risk that isincurred as a consequence, directly or indirectly, of the use and application of any of the contents of this work. Printed in the United Kingdom.

PAIN MANAGEMENT

for

CHRONIC BACK PAIN SUFFERERS

A GUIDE TO MANAGE CHRONIC LOW BACK PAIN SYMPTOMS

PROF. GEORGE ZAFIROPOULOS

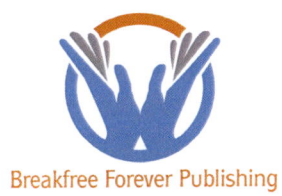

Breakfree Forever Publishing

IMPORTANT NOTICES / DISCLAIMERS

The depicted experience may not be considered as typical. Your background, education, experience and work ethic may differ. This is used as an example and not a guarantee of success. Individuals do not track the typicality of its student experiences. Your results may vary.

The contents of this training, such as text, graphics, images and other material, are intended for informational and educational purposes and not for the purpose of rendering medical or mental health advice. The contents of this training are not intended to substitute for professional medical advice, diagnosis and/or treatment. Please consult your medical professional before making changes to your diet, exercise routine, medical regimen, lifestyle, and/or mental health care.

This is not a medical consultation or medical advice. This is a guide to be followed, aiming to improve the quality of your life. You can keep all material that is necessary to you and discard what is not working for you.

Stories shared during the sessions of the modules are true experiences of me personally, or patients that have crossed paths with me during consultations many years ago. No personal details are shared within the course that will make them identifiable to anybody.

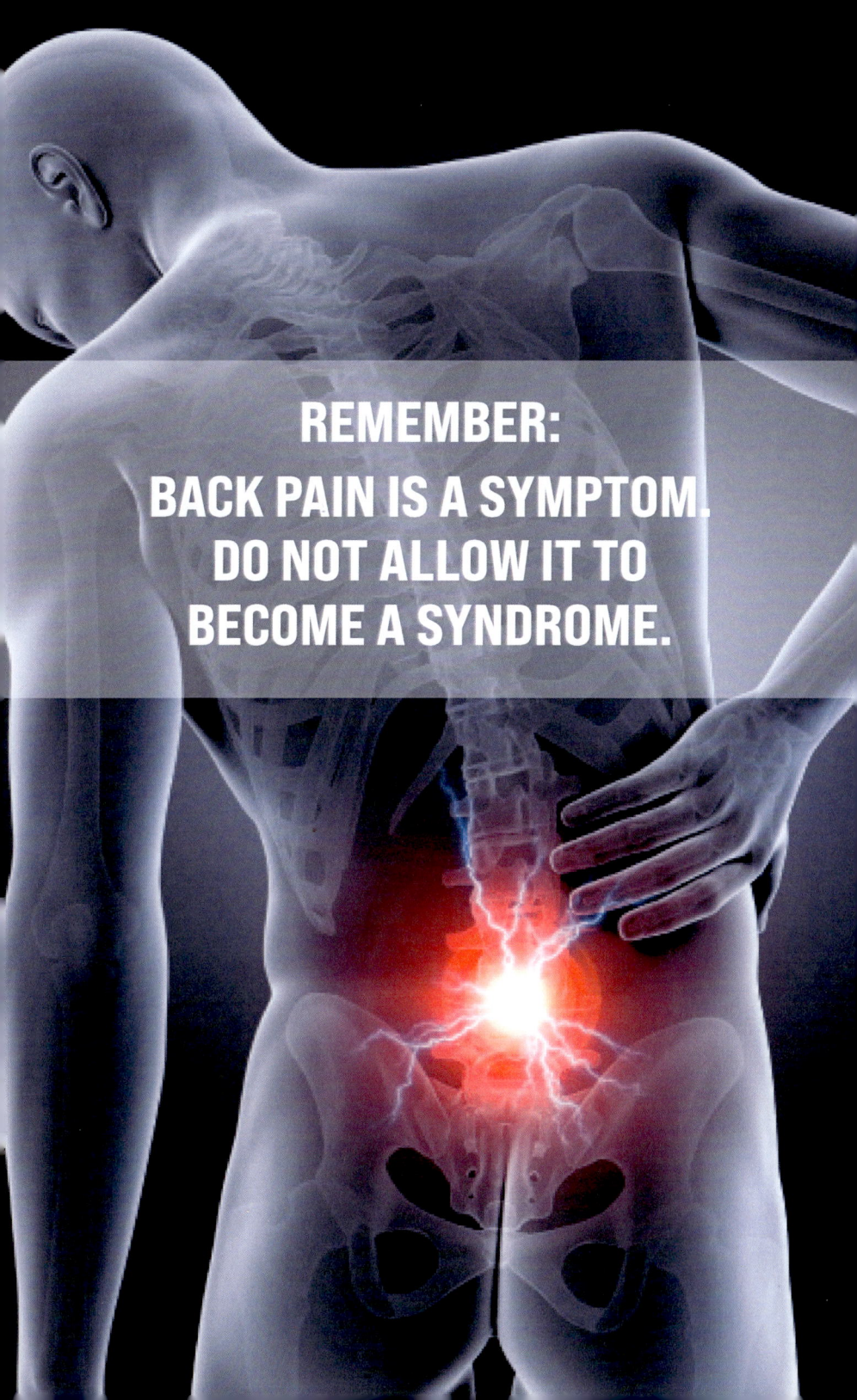

CONTENTS

Introduction 9

Science first 13
    Red flags 15
    The story 18

What is back pain? 25

Spinal Mechanism 35

How back pain affects people 49

"Chemical" effect 63

Doctor's understanding and limitations 67

Solution planning: 5 P's creating the 5 M's strategy 71
    Motion 81
    Music – Movies 83
    Meditation 86
    Mental awareness 88
    Marking down 93
    Recipes 102

Implementation 115
    Motion 117
    Exercises 121
    Music – Movies 160
    Meditation 161
    Breathing exercises 165
    Mental awareness 166
    Marking down 178

Epilogue 183
Evaluation 191

INTRODUCTION

In this book, I am encouraging you to go through the possible ways that can be used, so the effects of back pain (mainly chronic low back pain), would be reduced and lead to improvement of the quality of life for all suffering. Everybody who is a chronic low back pain sufferer can benefit from this book as there is a huge effect on their wellbeing. The professional as well as social life is affected, but mainly for those who are at the years of retirement and are missing the activities they may have with their loved ones and grandchildren.

This book has only educational purposes and cannot substitute the medical consultation, examination, and advice someone could receive from their family doctor.

Back pain is a very common problem that affects millions of people across the world. It is calculated that 9.4% of adults globally suffer from it. It is the second most common complaint that forces patients to go and visit their doctors and is related to musculoskeletal conditions. It is found that the effect on people who are in the productive age is enormous. Productivity of people at the age of 45 to 65 years old is reduced by 20% globally, although severe symptomatology can increase this to 43% reduction of working hours. This leads to financial loss. It is the most reported issue affecting adults over the age of 65 years old; an average of 22% in this category of people. Breaking this group in subgroups: back pain is present in 31% of people aged between 80 – 84 years old and 29% for those between 90 – 99 years old. In these groups, the pain takes on characteristics of disability in 6% and 10% respectively.

Someone could ask why one has to concentrate and offer educational material to these people who are in their golden years. What is the reason that such material cannot be in the hands of every person who is suffering from back pain? The answer is simple.

These senior citizens are a rapidly growing group - they are those who have the most common reported presentation of the symptoms and unfortunately are often excluded from any official clinical trial. I feel that they are the 'forgotten generation.' Again, the people could ask: "Really? Do we need to spend money and effort to study the problems of these old people?" And again, the answer would be simple. The 'old' people are those who spent their lives, time and effort to create the society others have the privilege to live in and on top of that, these 'old' people are, in the majority of the cases and in almost all countries of the world, those who take care of the younger generation, their grandchildren, as their parents are busy to go to work. In other words, the society is still depending upon these 'old' people and they are not here to be forgotten.

But who am I and what makes me qualified to talk about back pain?

I studied Medicine and later I specialised and became an Orthopaedic Surgeon. During my career, I have seen and treated a great number of people who have suffered with back pain, so I have some understanding about the condition, implications and effects of it in people's lives.

This is not the only fact that makes me able to talk about the condition. I was a severe chronic low back pain sufferer. This change was because I managed to find ways to control the constant low back pain and I live a much better life now.

Due to an injury I had in the past, I have been suffering with chronic low back pain and I know, well, what the meaning of 'back pain' is. While I was at the acute phase of my symptoms, I really wanted information, answers, and support, as I believe everyone wants when an illness hits them. I am close to my retirement age, so I can easily say that I am one of you in more than one level, for the following additional reasons. I am a chronic low back pain sufferer and old enough to understand all other limitations some of you have. On top of that, I have a total of over 42 years with medicine, science and experience on my side - 39 of those years within Orthopaedic surgery.

I would be humbled if you would allow me to share my experiences with you and assist your understanding of what low back pain is and how it is affecting us in the multitude of levels and systems of our body. The created material will drive us through the different pathways and step by step together, we will find the solution.

> **THIS IS NOT A MEDICAL CONSULTATION, BUT IT IS AN ADVENTURE THROUGH THE COLD CORRIDORS OF SCIENCE AND THE TUMULTUOUS WAYS OF THE MIND, AS BOTH BODY AND MIND SUFFER THE SAME FROM THIS CONDITION.**

SCIENCE FIRST

I know that the majority of you want to have answers, as you want to go back as quickly as possible and do your daily activities like your housework and even better take care of your grandchildren, the pride and joy of every family and the future of our society.

Unfortunately, though, you have to endure some scientific details and I will try to make them as simple as possible.

So, let us start with science.

Back pain is the symptom of a condition initially unknown and unclear, that affects our body. It extends from the shoulder blades to the small of our back and due to this spread we, as doctors, divide it to dorsal pain and low back pain, form a better understanding of the region we are talking about. In the present book, we will concentrate on low back pain. I repeat back pain is a symptom. If the back pain is present three months from the initial onset, then it is called chronic low back pain.

There are three common classifications of back pain:

1. Axial, called mechanical as well, and is present in a specific region.
2. Referred back pain, a dull pain irradiating to the back from a different area. It could be global (generalised pain) or localised to a specific area.

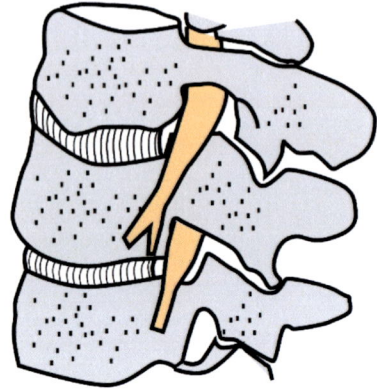

3. Radicular pain, when the pain is starting from the back and irradiates in the periphery following the route of the nerve which is irritated, mainly the lower leg.

In the present as already mentioned, we will concentrate on the chronic mechanical low back pain (localised at the lower part of the back).

> I HAVE TO STRESS THOUGH, THAT THIS MATERIAL HAS ONLY EDUCATIONAL PURPOSES. IT IS NOT PROVIDING ANY SPECIFIC MEDICAL OPINION TO SPECIFIC CONDITIONS AND TO SPECIFIC INDIVIDUALS. IT IS SERVING AS GUIDELINE FOR CHRONIC LOW BACK PAIN FOR THOSE PEOPLE WHO ARE NOT PRESENTING ANY RED FLAGS.

RED FLAGS

Red Flag: what is a **red flag**? It is the condition or symptom where if it is present to a person, this person has to visit their own doctor at their earliest convenience, because it could result in some unhappy consequences.

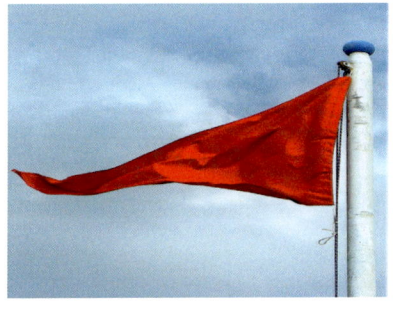

These are the most common red flags for a person presenting symptoms of back pain:

1. **Cauda equina syndrome**. In this condition there is 'saddle anaesthesia' present, meaning numbness or loss of sensation in the inner thighs, groins, gluteal region and perineum, loss of bladder or bowel control and weakness of the anal tone. This is an emergency.
2. **Spinal fracture**. This is the result of an injury. It could happen at any age, but for people above the age of 55, it could be presented as a sudden pain following a fall or minor injury on grounds of osteoporosis. It would be necessary to be investigated for the exclusion of the severity, pathology of the broken vertebra and possible further treatment would be necessary.
3. **Neoplastic deposits**. Usually these represent secondary deposits of a possibly already known primary malignancy. It is possible that the person may suffer from unexplained weight loss. Investigation, further opinion and possible treatment may be the course of action.
4. **Infection**. Pain appearing suddenly following a recent or even longstanding significant generalised infection. There is

the possibility of fever to accompany this pain. The condition has to be investigated and treated accordingly.

5. **Back pain associated with neurological symptoms**. Presentation of numbness or weakness of the legs, both or just the one. Further clinical evaluation would be necessary.
6. **Spinal stenosis**. Pain present in both legs after exercise, usually walking accompanied with mild numbness. The symptoms improve after the person either sits down, approximately the same time period as the time of walking or is leaning forward and supports self against a steady object. Following this period of immobilisation, the patient is able to walk again without or with minimum discomfort until the next forced, by the symptoms, stop.

> **FOR ALL OF THE ABOVE, YOU NEED TO SEE YOUR DOCTOR FOR FURTHER CONSULTATION, OPINION AND TREATMENT.**

Who am I? I am an Orthopaedic Surgeon close to retirement and I treated a lot of people with back pain throughout my career. But it is not only this that makes me able to talk about back pain. For the last 25 years, I have suffered from low back pain. I went through the symptoms that all low back pain sufferers go through and I came out a winner. I spent my entire life battling it. I had been swallowed by the dark canyon, but I fought and came back to light, climbing out of it at the opposite side.

I already mentioned briefly what makes me an authority on the field. I am one of the people who suffered from chronic low back pain and rarely still having the occasional symptoms, so I know exactly how people feel when they are hit by this. I lived all my working life suffering from this. On top of that. due to my professional position, for 43 years, I treated many who suffered with back pain symptomatology, so I am able to explain and make matters clearer to all.

I am here to offer my service to all, share my experiences and walk with all of you, step by step, the path that can lead all to 'freedom.' Freedom of the severe debilitating pain which demoralises all and drops us to the abyss.

But is freedom the complete elimination of your symptoms from your life? The answer is NO.

According to Pythagoras, the Greek philosopher, *"The person who is able to control self is free."*

In other words, freedom is the control of the symptoms; it is not the complete elimination. Finding ways of controlling and reducing the frequency and the time of suffering is a win and this is what all can call freedom.

THE STORY

For me, it all started one day in the operating theatre. I had to operate an acromegalic (giant in other words) patient. He was taller and longer than the operating table and his weight was more than 150 kilograms (330 pounds). After he was anaesthetised, we had to reposition and turn him to one side, in preparation for the operation.

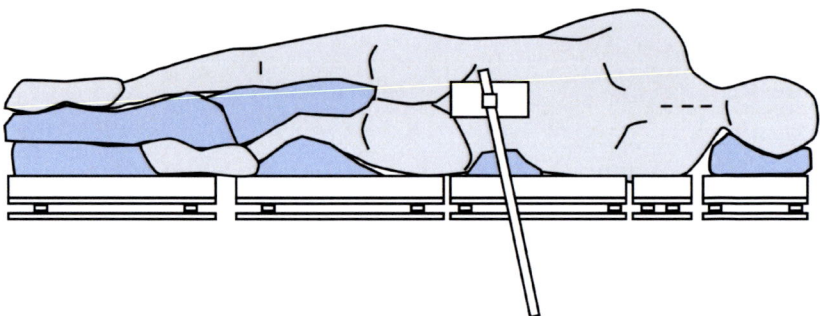

A team of six people gathered around the operating table, the anaesthetist on the top to control his head and neck, four people in one side to do the initial lifting and myself on the other side to help the lifting, pulling, finalising the position and eventually stabilising him with the necessary support. Unfortunately, during the final moment of countdown, a member of the team opposite to me, changed position resulting in the whole disorganisation of those who only sporadically lifted and I was left alone to pull almost 150kg on my own. My spine cracked and I felt pain running through the length of it. It took me sometime to straighten my body. I was given painkillers by one of the nurses and it took about half an hour to be able to come back to the upright position. I had to go ahead and perform the surgery, as there was no other surgeon available to help and after I finished the operation, I threw myself face down on one of the theatre trolleys. More painkillers were given to me and when I felt better, I drove home. That night I could not sleep, turning and tossing as I was trying to find a comfortable position. When I informed the hospital in the morning about my pain and stiff back, I was told that a clinic was already booked for me and they were unable to cancel it as there was nobody available to replace me, so I was called back on duty. This acute pain forced me to move in a tilted position. I went to my doctor who sent me plain X-rays and gave me painkillers. The results of the radiological investigations came as 'there is no congenital deformity or fracture,' something that I already knew. Following this, my doctor said that all of this was muscular - he was only providing me with painkillers and never sent me to physiotherapy or allowed me to stay out of duty.

The pain continued for months, and I was walking in pain, with a twisted back. My doctor was saying to me that I am an Orthopaedic Surgeon, so I knew how to treat back pains, and I had to ask myself about any treatment. On the subject there was a caveat; I could not self-refer to have any other treatment or investigation due to regulations and only he could offer such a service, by requesting or suggesting these alternatives.

About four or five months after that initial episode, another 'accident' made things better. I was dictating a letter to my secretary after a long day's work. My back pain was not permitting me to sit on my chair, so instead I placed my one knee on the seat and held the back of the chair to stabilise and rest from standing all day long. The chair was a rotating office seat and as I was talking, I suddenly lost balance and twisted my back trying to avoid a fall. A sharp pain went through my spine and this acute pain I had for months was gone. I was so happy, but over time I found out that it was replaced by a dull discomfort that became a constant presence. It was getting worse every morning. I had a stiff back, moving like a robot and with a lot of limitations, unable to bend freely in any direction. The pain had ups and downs in frequency and intensity throughout the day, but it was always present. This resulted to periodically using painkillers, helping me to cope with the symptoms. Physiotherapists in unofficial discussions, as I had not been referred to them, were not interested and as I had not presented any red flags and there was no appetite for any investigations, they thought that no treatment was necessary. My doctor was looking at me as a nuisance, so I stopped asking for help from him.

I chose to do the minimum movement and that resulted in a slow but steady increase of my weight. My mood was wavy, following my pain's frequency wave pattern, matching exactly the waves of the pain's intensity. When my pain was increasing, my mood was decreasing and the opposite. Family life was affected because of my behaviour. Nobody was happy anymore. Everybody was under stress. I was constantly worried and questioning whether this would be my life from that time onwards and I believe the rest of the family had the same thoughts, but they were not voicing them. I was getting deeper and deeper into depression, driving everybody around me to the same dark place. In addition, my general health started to be influenced by the whole condition. I was not able to climb stairs anymore, I had lost stamina, I was getting breathless, and my blood pressure went through the roof. I was worrying about myself, but I also had to look after my patients, adding extra stress on me.

One day, my doctor called me and said that I may be close to a pre-diabetic status and he only wanted to 'feed' me more pills, of all kinds, to control my 'issues.' This treatment had to be for life. That was the wakeup call. Something kicked in my brain. I was not prepared to keep taking medications for life. When I refused his offer, he looked at me and gave me an ultimatum of six months to pull myself out of my misery. I had to change my body and my attitude within this given time. I was in the depth of a dark valley and I had to come out of it. I had to be resurrected by becoming free from all these troubles that had crossed my path and threw me into the abyss.

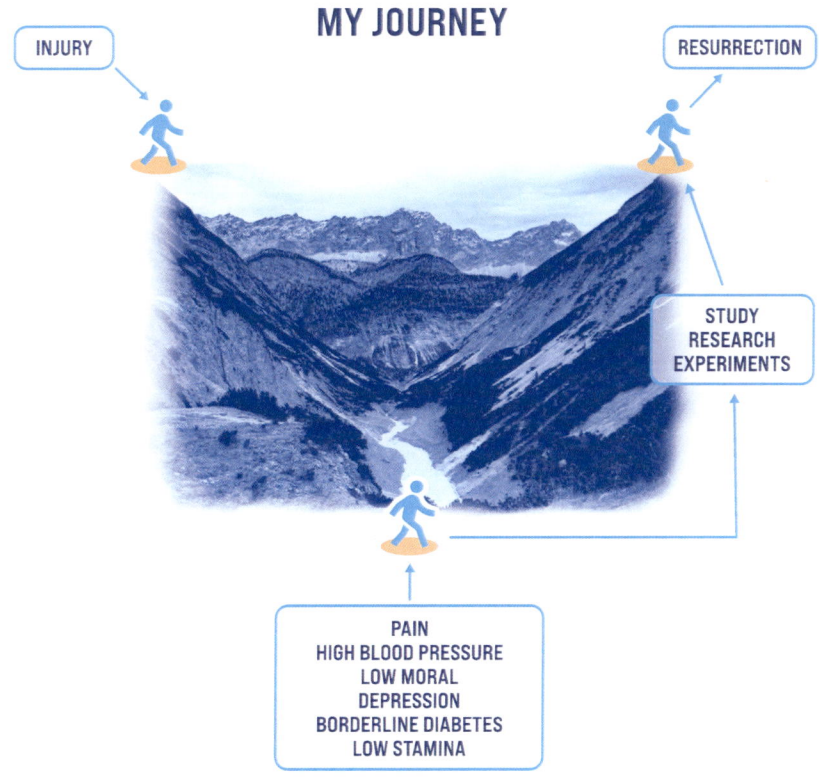

That was it. I started my own research, and I studied numerous papers and books. As nobody was prepared to help me, I had to help myself. I went back to be reminded about metabolism in the physiology textbook, endocrinology and finally chronic pain management. Following all this, with a lot of trial and error, I successfully done it.

Initially, I started to move. The short walks became longer and slowly, I could walk miles on miles. I joined the gym, lost weight. Blood pressure and blood sugar went back to normal levels and as my body became stronger, my dull back pain was visiting me on rare occasions. My mood swings stopped, I became happier, and my family started to smile again. Saying all that, I stress to all of you, that I know what chronic back pain is. I went through it and conquered it.

Having this life experience and being able to understand the situation having the professional and scientific knowledge, I am able to help others to overcome the same problems by sharing the information and support, something that nobody provided to me when I needed it. I am ready to talk about the steps and strategies that helped me to get through this burden.

I look forward to this challenge; I am ready to serve my senior retired folks who are suffering from chronic mechanical back pain, to understand their back pain and achieve an improvement of the quality of their life. I want you to be active again, to be able to play with your grandkids, be able to take care of yourselves and do what back pain stopped you from doing.

This is my purpose: to help you move forward; to help you to come out of the misery back pain is forcing you to live through and to help you to control your symptoms. As mentioned, by controlling them, you will become free.

To do this, you need to learn about back pain. Education on this subject is necessary and I am here and prepared to help you understand back pain.

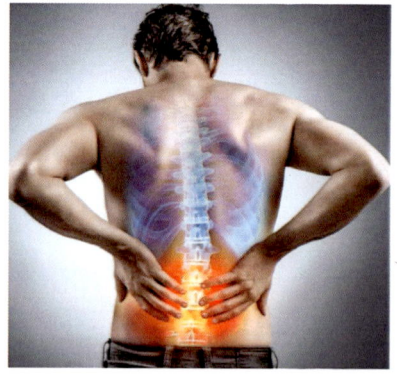

In the following chapters there will be some more science; unfortunately, it's necessary, but it will be presented in simple enough ways. You will read about the common causes and symptoms back pain has and what back pain is, but I will go deeper when explaining this. I will be trying to present to you the way back pain can affect people on physical, mental and social levels, what steps and strategies you can use to resolve the symptoms and how these strategies can be planned and implemented.

> **I MUST REPEAT, THIS IS NOT A MEDICAL CONSULTATION AND SOME STRATEGIES MAY NOT BE SUITABLE FOR YOU. TAKE WHAT SUITS YOU AND THROW AWAY THE REST.**

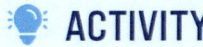
ACTIVITY

Please reflect and write:

1. How long have you been suffering from back pain?
2. How was this back pain presented to you?
3. What have you done to improve it?
4. What is your current state?

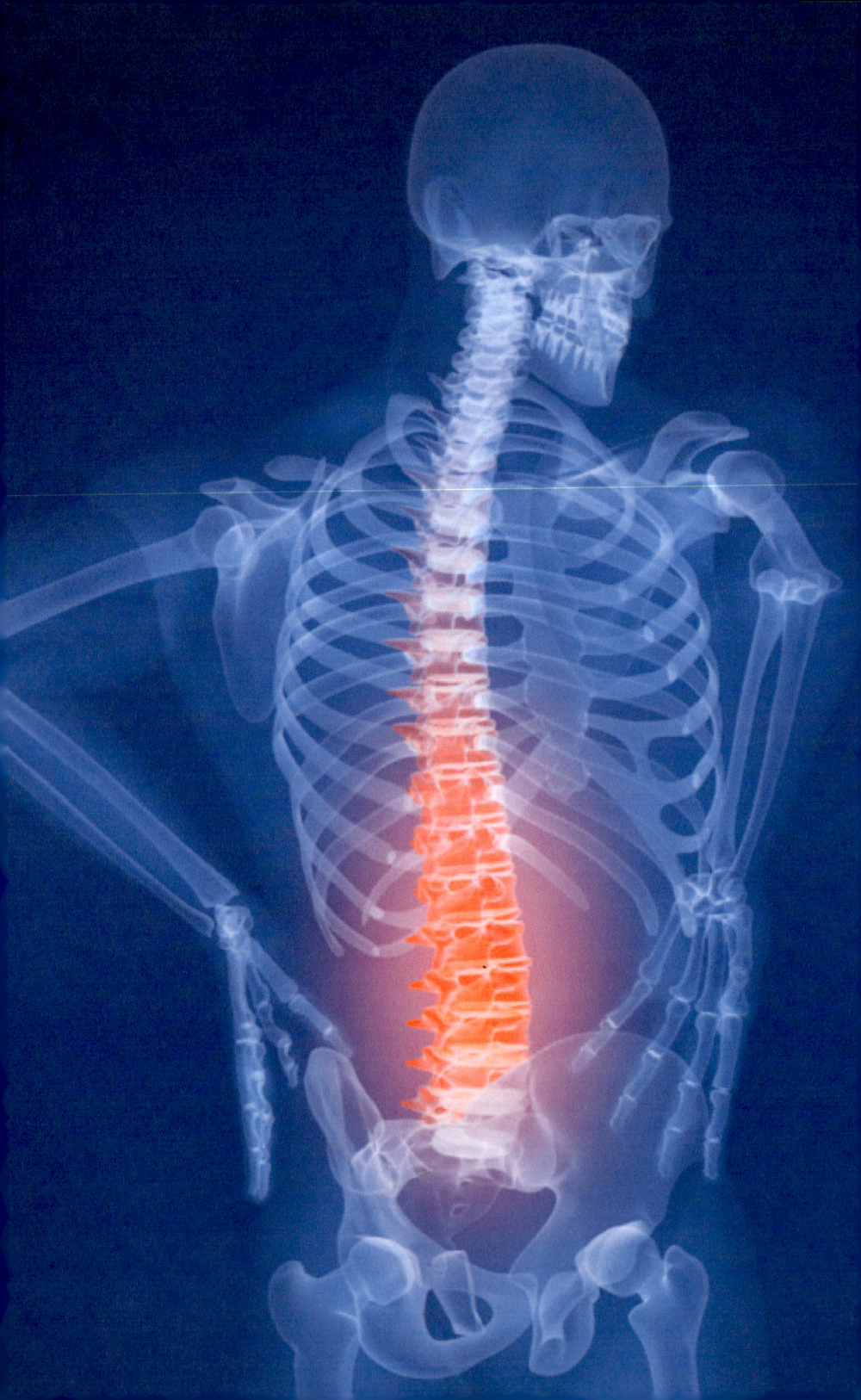

WHAT IS BACK PAIN?

We all know what back pain is, as we have experience of it, but do we really know it?

Physically, it is a pain present in our back; most of the times at the small of the back and can spread in both your buttocks, having the feeling of a heavy load or sometimes characteristics of dull or even sharp squeezes at the area like a vice. Other times, it presents itself like a broad belt, starting at the centre of our lower back, spreading to our side, involving our core from the ribs down.

There are times it also appears as a sharp stab feeling, that can take your breath away, causing you to look like a surprised person who does not understand where this lightning bolt came from. But other times, it can be deceiving and can be represented as a 'sweet' stiffness that stops any movement of the body. It may seem like a tooth of a gear came out of place (from the existing 'gears' of your body machine), and you start rotating, bending and twisting in your attempt to put it back in place, so you will be able to continue the motion you had initially started.

In addition to all this, there are times when the pain spreads well beyond the buttocks towards the sides of the hips, or down to the leg or both legs. Even this can vary. It can be a niggling or sharp pain with the presence of numbness of part of the leg or it can spread to both. It can be there constantly, or it can come up only after we had

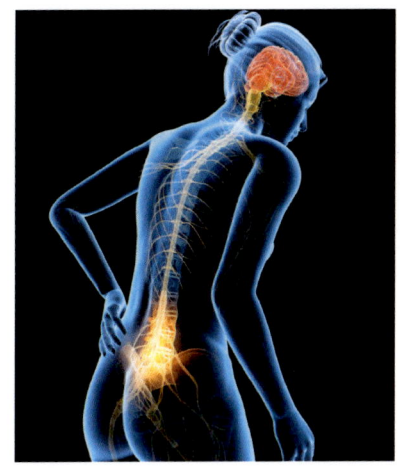

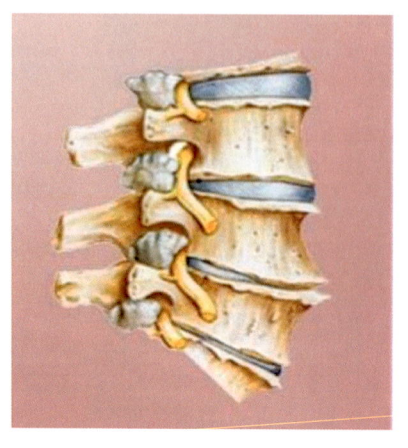

walked for some time. This latter symptomatology can force you to stop and sit on a bench for almost the same amount of time you walked, so you can enjoy the surroundings or the sunset. Or it can make you bend and lean forward to the nearby existing railing of the neighbour's fence and try to make friends with the dog that is roaming in the front garden. There are though, these scary moments when the pain and numbness are so severe that you may lose control of your body functions, and you may lose your dignity this way, ending up wet and dirty not knowing how all this happened. This fills fear in your hearts. The described main symptomatology is this of spinal stenosis, although the latter symptoms present neurological dysfunction, due to pressure on spinal cord. Within the above paragraphs, some described symptoms may also be present when a red flag exists.

These are the majority and most frequent presentations back pain takes and people are suffering from. These symptoms are described as representations of a 'monster,' that is there to torture them and make their life miserable. But do not forget that back pain is a symptom, not a diagnosis.

As I explained, the present book is concentrating on the mechanical back pain; we ignore any pain with neurological symptoms.

In my case, the morning inability to move freely and come out of bed was the main problem for months. Every morning at the initial stages, I had to be assisted by my wife to pull me out of bed. My moral was very low. My family was stressed to the upper limit. I could 'participate' at the dinner table only by standing. It was eating like I was at a fast-food café and straight after that, I was running to hide in my corner. I stopped communicating and withdrew into myself, like a tortoise in its shell. I knew that my spinal roots and nerves were not affected, but I did not want to live such a life.

What was the mechanism forcing me to act like this?

In the following paragraphs, you will see the effect of chronic back pain and the mechanical function of the spine.

The presenting physical symptom of someone who is suffering from low back pain at the initial stages, is restriction of mobility. This affects the everyday activities this person can perform, either at home or work. For the majority of you, work is not an issue as you are retired, but for those who are still working because you are near to retirement or those who have other activities and hobbies, lack of mobility is a problem. At the same time, emotions are flooding your brain and that affects you more. This is the time when we all need to know what is happening and need guidance as well as education to learn about back pain, how to modify your activities and how to continue your physical activities.

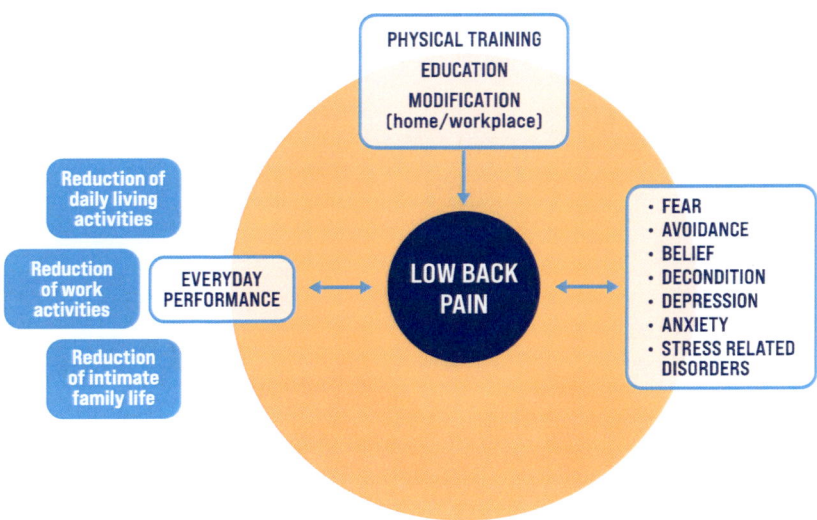

From the diagram above it is obvious that the mechanical low back pain at the initial stages has an effect on the daily activities but also puts a great weight to another "sphere" of your Existence and the emotions create fear and a multitude of more severe emotional presentation.

Initially, I thought that physical education and training had not been affected by the emotional sphere. This is not really true. It is affected and can affect the emotions back.

What mechanisms is the body going through though?

By only hearing the words 'back pain,' your brain goes to full alert, your mind fills with fear and your breathing becomes quicker as adrenaline and cortisol flow uncontrollably in your arteries, trying to make you run and flee from monster's grip. As you find out, you cannot. You cannot because the back is not leaving you, as it threw the chains around your body and is holding you captive.

It is at that moment when your mental reaction is creating more problems to you. The whole story starts with the reaction of your primary brain; this is part of your brain. It kicks in and the escape mechanisms influence your developed brain. These mechanisms trigger more fear and anxiety, and your emotions now cloud your mind, and the panic reaction starts, like a fish out of water. Your mind screams of despair and does not allow any rational thoughts, as your emotions flood your full existence. You cannot comprehend how and why this is happening to you.

One thing though, it is obvious. With physiotherapy and movement, as well as education and some modifications in your daily mobility, there is a strong possibility that it will be controlled at these early stages. It is possible this way to overcome the emotional burden, as movement is giving you confidence and confidence makes you happy. So movement can affect your emotions as shown in the diagram.

On the other hand, when back pain is present for more than three months, then it is considered as chronic and the reaction is a bit different.

The initial cause of the pain could be the same or different to the one in the acute phase, but there is a greater influence on your mental status, as even your social life is influenced. This is where the quality of your life is affected.

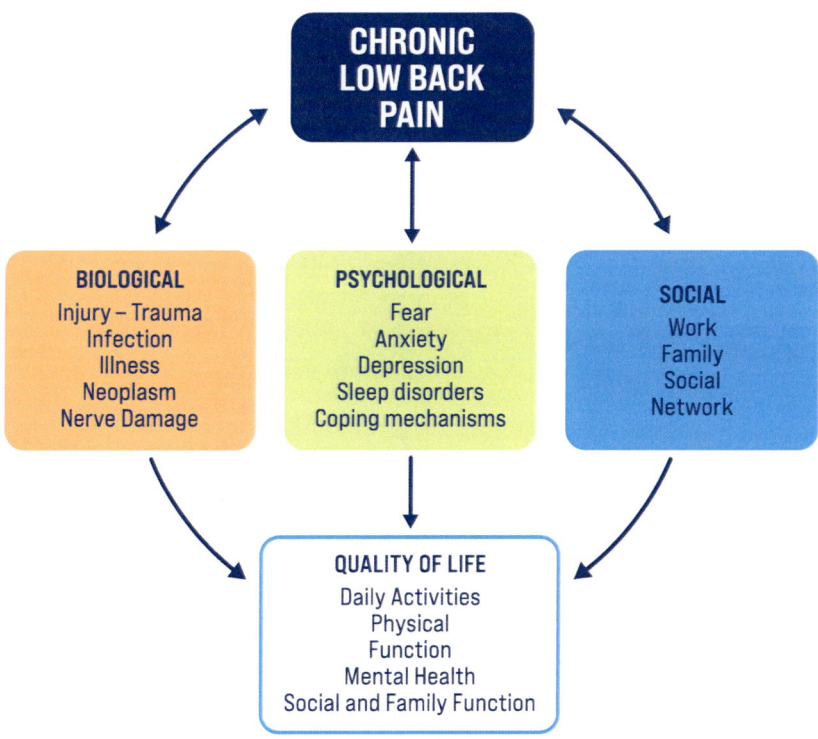

From this diagram, someone can observe that chronic low back pain has an indirect effect on the quality of your life. By affecting your psychology and social life, it places a heavy load on you. The physical as well as the psycho-social issues can fuel the back pain, and this is a non-stop cycle. There is also a direct influence between these three parts. You live a life full of frustration, disappointment, and despair. All this is much better illustrated in the diagram below.

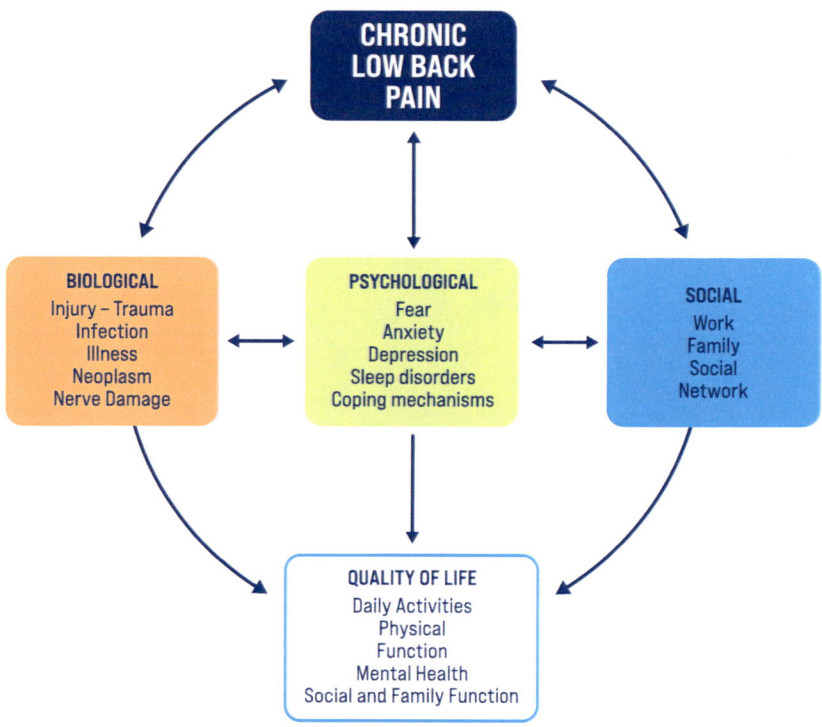

There is though, a theoretical question.

Is back pain your enemy, as you may think or is it your Friend?

Do not forget that back pain is a symptom, not a diagnosis.

You may have had the injury years ago and the symptoms may have settled, but now you have pain again. Why did it present itself again now and not two or three years ago? What is the reason?

Do you need to fight it or learn what it is and be able to live with it, in the same way that you learn to live with your new neighbour who has a hyperactive child?

You all know the story of Dennis, nicknamed 'Dennis the Menace,' who initially annoyed the elderly man living next to his house with 'inappropriate activities.' At the end, he became a valuable friend. Can you call back pain a friend? This is a matter of opinion.

It depends on the prospective angle you see it from. If you see it as an enemy and nothing else, then you have to fight it. You know that fights create injuries in both parties. On the other hand, 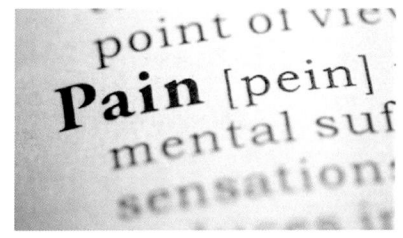 if it is a friend, why is it creating these horrible symptoms and why are you suffering? There is the possibility that it is trying to protect you from movements that can create more damage to your body. You must not forget that most of the time, the mechanical back pain is linked with an injury that happened in the past, either acutely or through a repetitive stressful action. During the initial stages, you brace yourself and try to heal the underlying cause. Back pain seems to be a defensive mechanism of your body. Analysing it further, back pain is a symptom and not the condition itself. The problem is that you take this symptom, feed it to your brain and make it swell with fear, resulting in a continuum of bracing, muscle spasms and secondary functional pains. This way, you are driving yourselves to the chronic low back pain and the continuous suffering. You make a symptom turn into a syndrome.

What creates the back pain?

Some of the causes of back pain according to literature are:

BIOLOGICAL	OCCUPATIONAL ACTIVITIES	MENTAL HEALTH ISSUES	NON-DIRECT SPINAL CONDITION
Injury/strain resulting to muscle, ligament, disc or bone tissue damage	Bad posture/ positioning	Sleeping disorders	Smoking
Degeneration of the tissues	Bad physical exercise	Depression	Pregnancy
Structural problems / Abnormal curvatures	Poor physical fitness	Anxiety	Shingles
High BMI (Body Mass Index)	Sedentary lifestyle		Kidney disease
Osteoporosis			Menstrual circle
Age			

In the diagram below you can observe that spinal loading is higher when you are sitting than when you are standing straight.

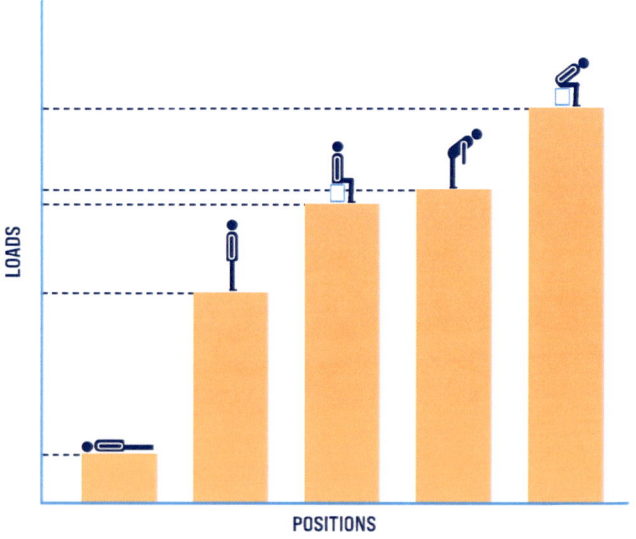

So my friends just sit back, calm down and enjoy the ride on your journey of learning how to live with your back pain as a friend and not an enemy.

 WE NEED TO LEARN:
1. How the spine works.
2. What can make the pain increase.
3. How we can approach this issue that knocked on our door.

SPINAL MECHANISM

Spine and mainly the neural system (central nerves and brain) are the first structures that are created in our embryonic life. Fully developed, the spine is made from a series of 'cylindrical' type bones called vertebrae, linked between them like a bicycle chain. Behind these cylindrical bones there are some arches and they are linked one over the other, creating a tube, the spinal canal. Within it, for most of the spine's length runs the spinal cord, which is nerve tissue and a continuation of our brain. At the lower levels of this spinal tube and at the end of the cord, we have only nerve roots inside the canal. Due to their appearance, we call them *cauda equina*, which in Latin means horse tail; this is what they look like. Along the spine cord, we have nerve roots that are coming out of the canal in every level and as soon as they come out, they link between themselves in the different levels creating the peripheral nerves, which run throughout the body.

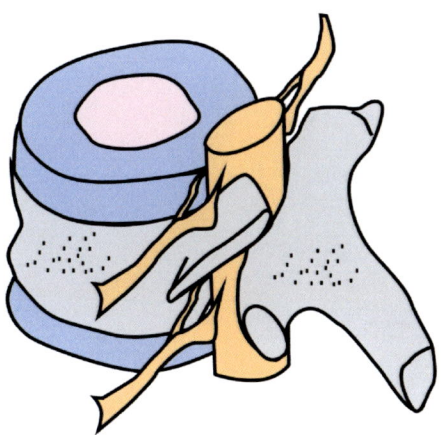

The spine, if we see it from the front is straight for its entire length, but if we see it from the side is curved. There are four different curvatures, two curving forward and two backward. The neck and lower back part, lean backwards and the dorsal and sacral area forwards. The forward curves called kyphotic and the backward lordotic. These names may help you to understand the terminology in case you read a report from an investigation you have done.

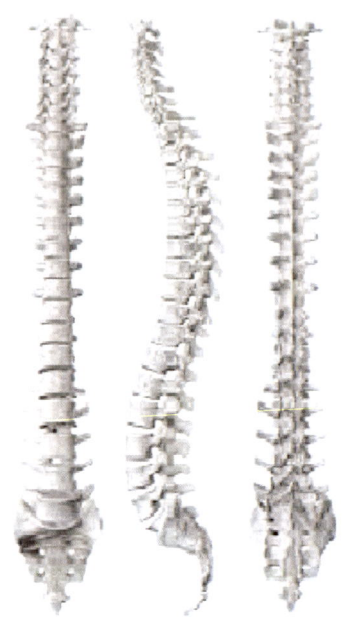

The vertebrae are linked between them with joints, which are part of the arch, called facet joints and ligaments that run in front, as well as the sides of the vertebrae. The joints are covered by their capsule and their own ligaments.

Between the vertebrae in each level we have another fixture, the intervertebral disc. Discs are made mainly from two parts. An elastic but firm ring, called annulus and a central jelly type substance, called nucleus. The latter is under tension within the whole structure.

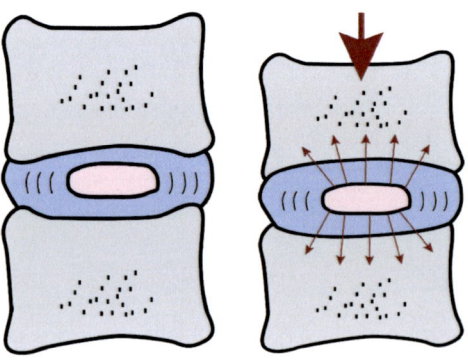

In the diagrams above, it is evident how the nucleus that is under tension is reacting when it is loaded.

If we examine the mechanical properties of the disc, we will discover, in its simplicity, that it is nothing more than a shock absorber.

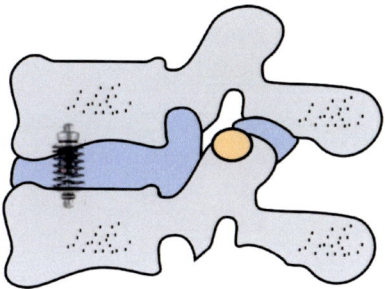

Annulus is made from layers and layers of rings – more or less similar structure to an onion.

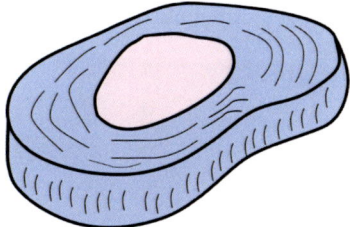 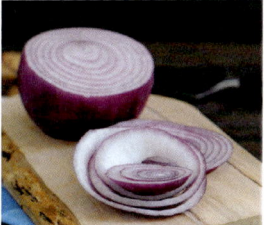

The only difference between the two, except the shape and the smell, is the direction of the fibres in each one of the layers. In the onion, the fibres of each layer are parallel running from the root to stem and this pattern is observed in all layers.

In the disc, the fibres of each layer are parallel in each layer, like the onion, but the direction differs between neighbouring layers. If one has an oblique direction from right to left, the one next to it will have direction from north to south (north the head, south the feet) and the third oblique from left to right and so on. This way, the sum of all layers creates a strong net and this strength is kept intact at all times even if the body is rotated.

This is because the different layers rotate accordingly and for example, the one that was running from north to south in a rotation may run obliquely from right to left and the neighbouring changes accordingly. This is giving the same strength to annulus in all potential positions the body takes and protects the nucleus in the same position and with the same properties.

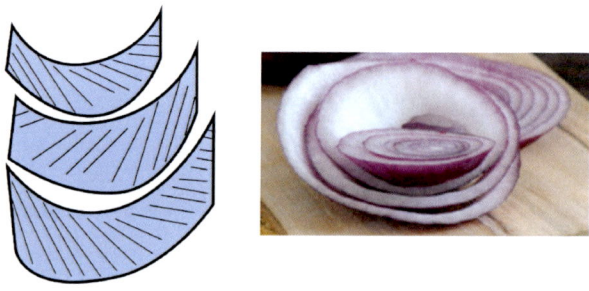

Unfortunately, as time goes by and with the use, or to put it better, misuse of the spine, the whole disc structure can become dehydrated. In this case, the 'selfish' nucleus sucks fluid from the neighbouring annulus, in the attempt to keep the shock absorption properties. This way, the annulus becomes drier and more fragile.

In this case, if an unusually excessive mechanical stress is applied to the back, the annulus may break, and the under-tension disc will protrude into the canal where the cord and the roots exist. Depending on the amount of disc displacement and the severity of pressure applied on the nerves, there may be neurological symptoms. There are also times that this disc dehydration is gradual and the space between the vertebrae under the body's weight becomes smaller. In these cases, they are reported as 'degenerated discs.'

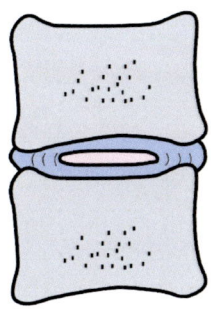 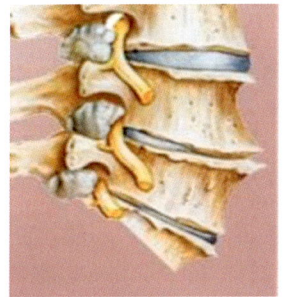

In the above diagram, the degenerative bulging disc where the nucleus became narrower and lost height, is illustrated, resulting in bulging discs, showing the disc as a deflated car tyre.

In the photo next to it, there is an artistic representation of narrow intervertebral spaces with formation of osteophytes (extra bone 'spikes') at the superior and inferior parts of the vertebrae.

This latter picture indicates degeneration of the disc and the spine in general.

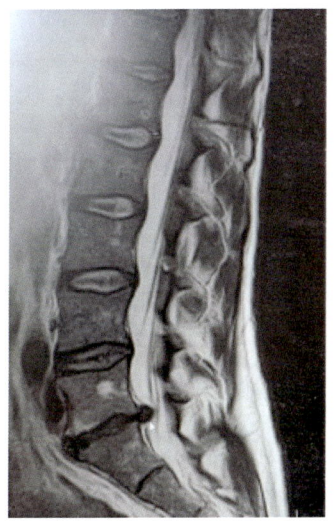 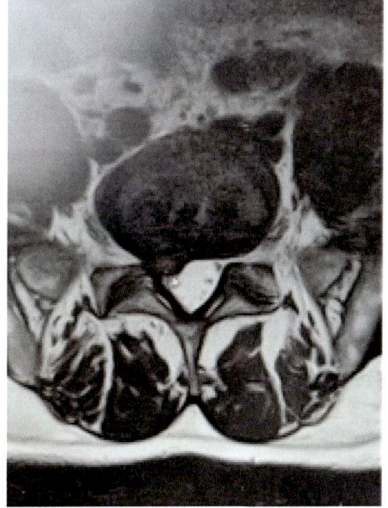

In the cases when the disc is degenerative and bulging, meaning that it has lost height, there is an effect on the facet joint position, which now are 'subluxed' (meaning that they are not in their ideal position), resulting to 'arthritic' changes, as they are 'grinding' their surfaces in these new positions. Think of these surfaces as two milestones that are slightly displaced and have to match their surfaces again. This procedure though, creates some inflammation in the area.

On the other hand, the scan on the right shows how the nucleus of the disc is penetrating to the left, after breaking the annulus and pressing on the cord and possibly one of the roots.

Despite all this, not all the loads were absorbed by the bones and discs, but the muscles play a very significant role to this offloading. They are not only there to move the bones, but also to support them. These muscles on their own can be considered as additional shock absorbers. Think of them as sacks of fluid that are hermitically closed and that there is the ability to change the viscosity of this fluid. The higher the viscosity, the more resistance of the structure exists. In other words, the stronger the muscle is, the more load it can take on, something that anyone agrees with.

On top of that, the most important structure is a network of veins that exists all around the spinal cord and penetrates the bones. This network of veins is called the *Plexus of Batson*, as he was the one who described 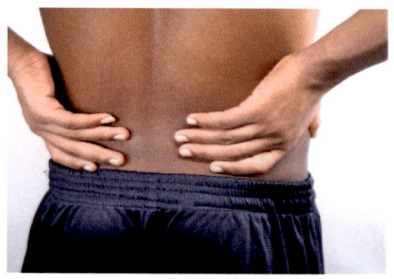 them. It is linked with the inferior veins that exist in the abdomen and the superior veins that exist in the thoracic cavity (chest).

These veins don't have valves like other veins in our body. If we increase the intra-abdominal or intra-thoracic pressure, blood is driven to these veins and the flow can be from either direction.

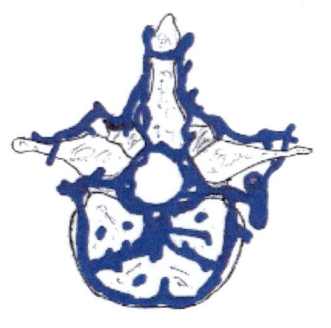

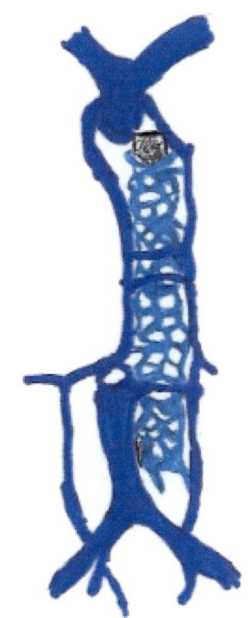

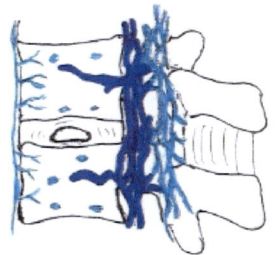

These diagrams show how the lower and higher main body veins are linked via this network of the *Plexus of Batson* and how this network is penetrating the bones.

The mechanical properties of this network can be very easily explained, if the mechanism that is used for lifting heavy objects is explained.

Just picture a heavyweight lifting athlete in the Olympic Games and track the movements and actions he or she does in preparation. You will observe that as soon as they call him/her and after she/he powders the hands, the intra-abdominal pressure is increased when he/she tightens her/his belt very tight. Then while he/she is preparing to

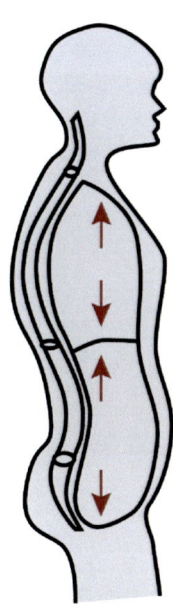

lift, a deep breath is taken and he/she holds the air in. This way the intra-thoracic pressure is increased. By doing this, the diaphragm (a muscle that separates the chest from the abdomen), is immobilised as well, under the pressure in both cavities. There is similar action at the pelvic floor; (incidental note: weak pelvic floor muscles can lead to bladder leak in case of weight lift).

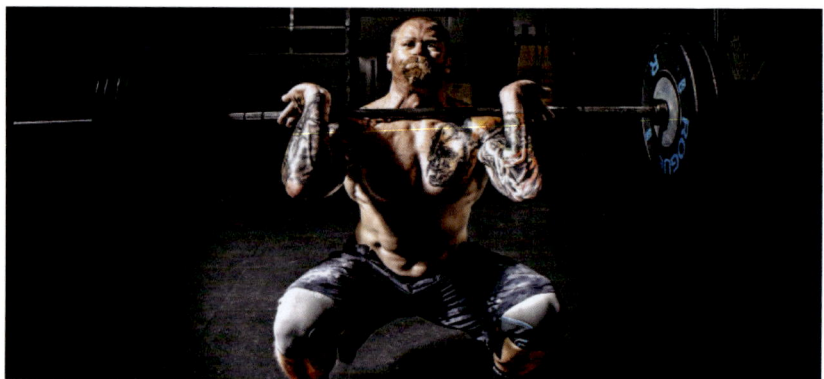

You can see in this picture how the veins around his neck are more prominent; this is due to the increased intrathoracic pressure.

It is obvious how the athlete is holding his breath in the attempt to hold the weight over his head.

At the end of the successful lifting, action and while the weights are lowered, a cry comes out of the mouth. This cry is a violent exhale of the held in air.

You may ask though, what is the reason I am going through this? It is simple. With all these actions, the athlete had pushed a vast amount of blood through this venous network, the *Plexus of Batson*, from both directions, abdomen and chest and really the whole lifting was done by using a hydrostatic pressure mechanism assisted by lever mechanism. It is the same way a heavy truck is lifted at the side of the road to change a flat tyre. Usually a hydraulic jack is used in comparison with the means used to lift a sedan, where a jack that is made by arms and hinges (applying mechanical lever mechanism principles) is used, because the car is lighter than the truck.

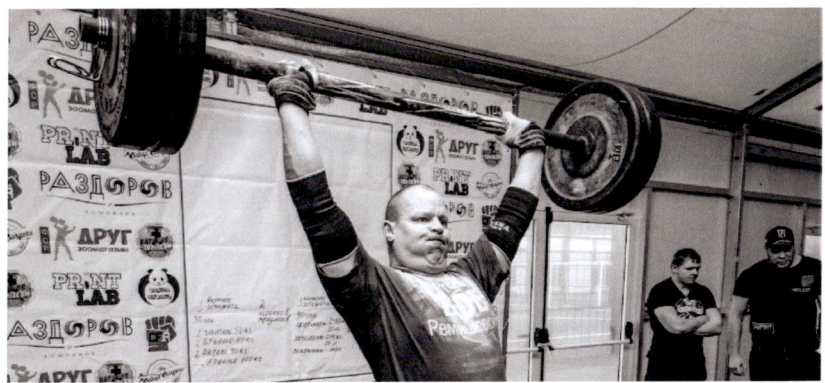

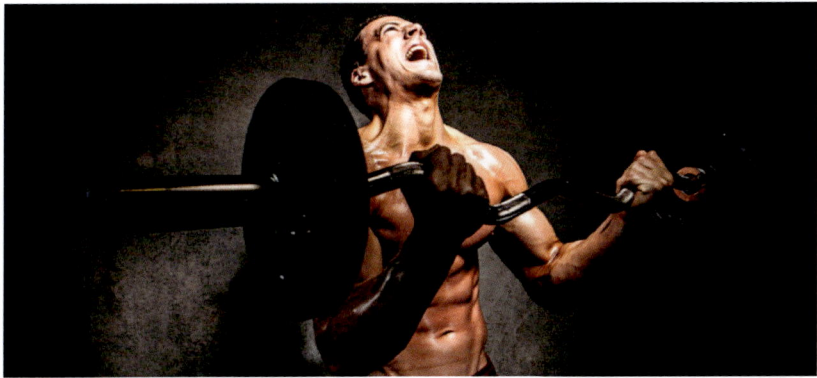

The human body (as it is obvious by these athletes), can lift a great deal of weight. The majority of people are not aware of the exact number of loads that can go through our body every day during our daily activities. The forces that are applied on our muscles and joints are of a scale that sometimes the mind is not able to comprehend.

There are a number of scientists that went through and measured the loads that can go through the different parts of the body - this part of science is called Biomechanics.

Measuring the forces that they take to go through our spine, you will be surprised. An experiment was done trying to calculate the loads going through our lower back. They used an individual of average weight and height and a weight of **20**kg. This weight was positioned in different places and was lifted in different ways. When the weight was placed in front of the individual's feet and asked to bend and lift it, they calculated that the load through the lower back was equivalent to **26**kg. If the weight from the same position was lifted after they asked the individual to bend their knees and reach it with a straighter back, the load was calculated to be **15**kg. Then, they moved the weight in an arm's length position on a lower height and lifting was ordered with extended arm if possible. The calculated load was equivalent to **480**kg.

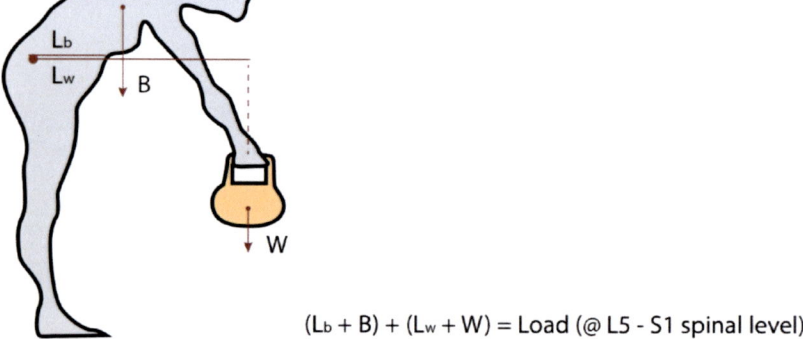

$(L_b + B) + (L_w + W) = $ Load (@ L5 - S1 spinal level)

Thinking of the daily activities that anyone executes, this latter position is used so many times during the day. For example, when a mother is trying to save her child by lifting it from the ground, while the kid is running towards the stairs, or the cook is lifting the pot full of water from the back burner of the stove. In all these actions, a very high load is placed on the spine and then everyone wonders why he/she ends up with back pains.

Then someone has to consider their own somatotype. The width of the body (if it is observed from the side), plays a role on the load put through the spine. The wider the body, the longer the imaginary moment arm on which the body weight is applied, while someone is in a standing position. This results in a greater force being applied to the muscles around the spine, particularly the posterior muscles.

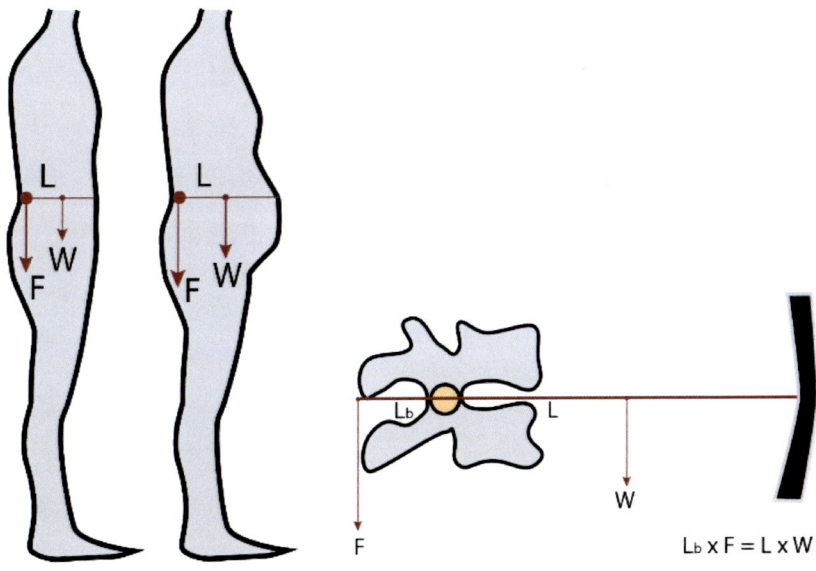

$$L_b \times F = L \times W$$

This is evident in the diagrams shown above and how the forces can be calculated. The equation is simplified to the extreme as other forces that can be applied on the body are not represented on the equation itself. The wider the body, the higher the force used to keep us upright. In the case of much wider body structure, the vector of the weight is moving forwards. If the example of a pregnant woman is used, the vector representing the weight can move considerably in front of the base of the body, (in other words in front of the feet and so there could be the tendency to topple the body forwards). That is the reason why a pregnant woman's standing position changes, by hyperextending her spine (bending backwards), allowing her to stabilise herself as she stands.

Finally, discs are shock absorbers, but our muscles have shock absorbing properties. Therefore, stronger muscles can relieve strain on the spine and address the role of viscosity differences mentioned above.

The shape and function of the spine can be influenced by other body pathologies. Hip problems, such as arthritis and stiffness of the joint, can make the symptoms of back pain more obvious because of one muscle that links the leg directly with the pelvis and the spine, at the same time.

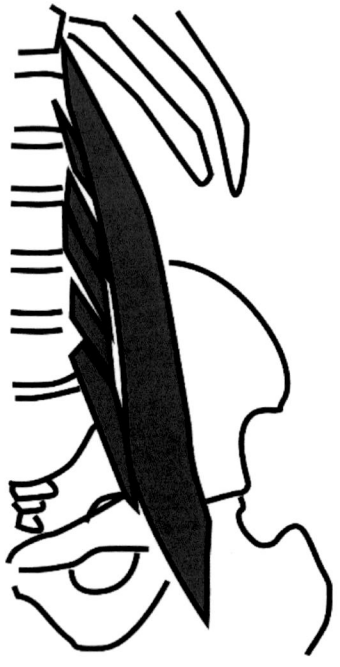

This muscle is called Iliopsoas and is a combination of two muscles with different initial origin but common attachment. These muscles are *Iliacus*, its belly is found at the inner side of pelvis and *Psoas*, its belly is attached in the small lateral processes and bodies of the lower vertebrae. Both bellies come to a united attachment with a common tendon, at the inner side of the femur (thigh bone) close to the hip joint. Someone could simplistically say that this muscle is linking the spine to the leg.

In the case of hip joint arthritis, the muscle could be stiffened and shortened in the attempt to protect and prevent the extreme movements of the hip joint. This way it is pulling the spine forward and has, as result, a crucial role to the spinal loading. In the case of an individual suffering from back pain, there is functional change of the spine and potential increase of the symptoms.

In summary, simple mechanical chronic back pain can be the result of one or many different causes that can affect a person. Understanding the mechanisms and function of our spine can help us to comprehend our condition and we could reflect by going deep to find out what initiated our individual issue and how we can approach it in the future.

> 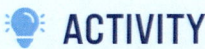 **ACTIVITY**
>
> Reflect and write down:
> 1. What was/is causing or making your back pain worse, in your opinion?
> 2. What remedies have you used to improve your symptoms?

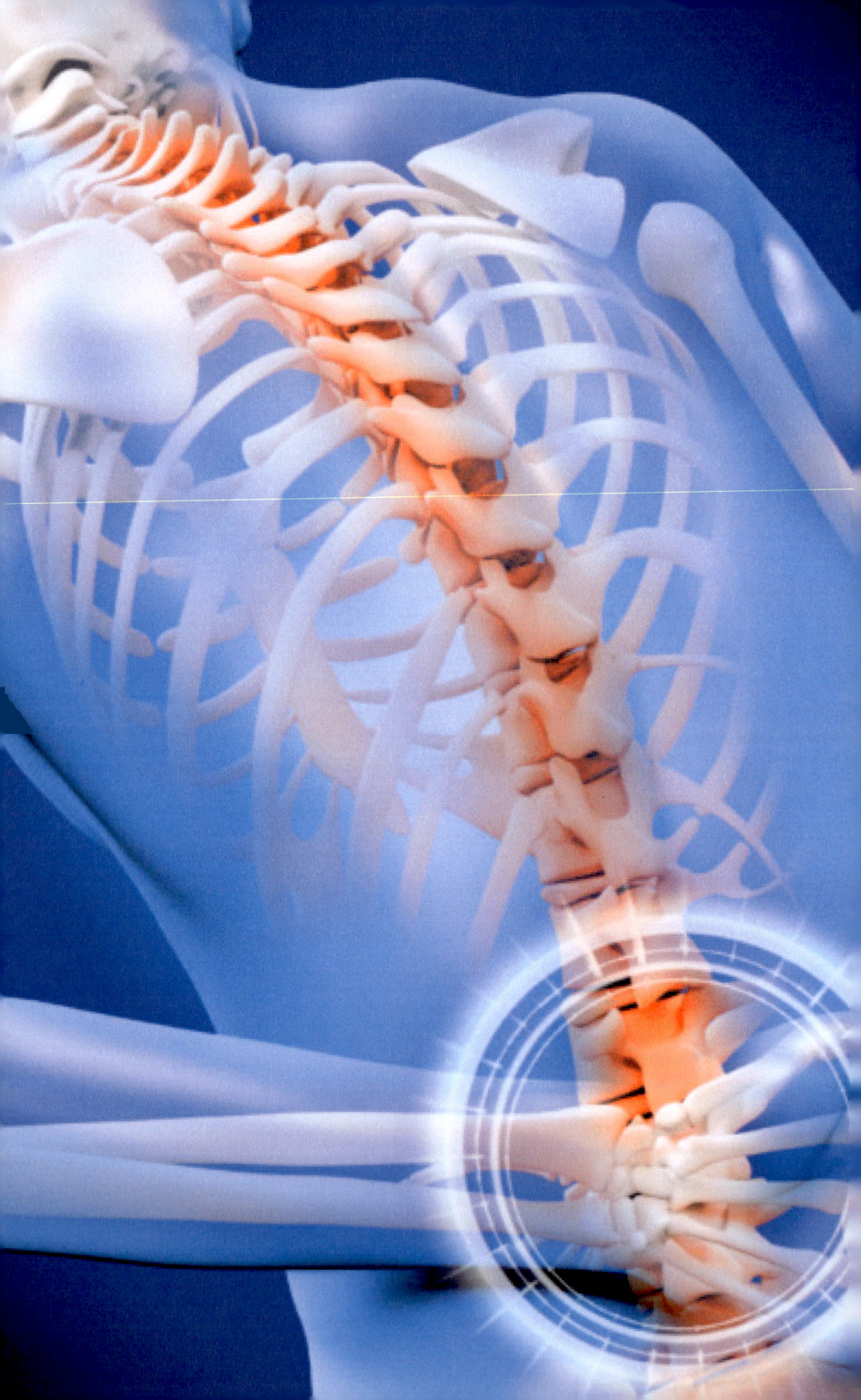

HOW BACK PAIN AFFECTS PEOPLE

When back pain hits you, the physical trauma or tissue damage, as in every case of trauma, is affecting your whole body. There is this alarm that rings up in the brain, causing it to try and understand what is happening. Emergency measures are called to be taken in place and different channels of different functions are disrupted.

The only channel that works is self-preservation. The picture you are taking is the same of a traumatised animal, isolating itself in the nest; the same action is taken by humans.

The first thing you do is to go to your safe corner and keep quiet. You don't want anyone to come and approach you. You don't want to move; you don't want to talk and you only want to be isolated. In other words, you want to find out what is happening, analyse and understand the situation, before thinking and planning the next steps you need to take.

This latter is also the issue. Are you able to make the correct decision and act accordingly or not?

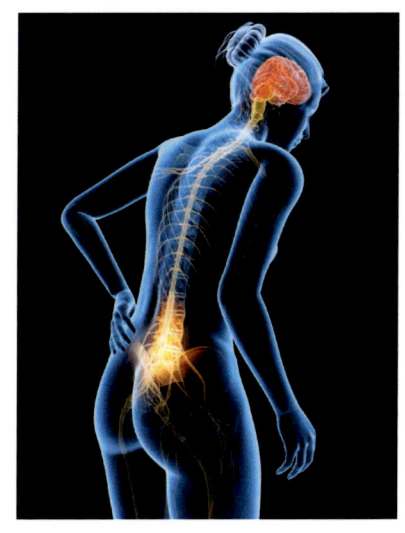

A number of questions have to be answered. These questions are mainly products of your own brain. They are thoughts that are coming through the channels of previous painful experiences - they are flashing back and you are trying to put them in place.

You analyse the condition under your own perspective. This may be confusing and potentially wrong.

Some more questions may come from your environment, your loved ones, your extended family, your friends, your co-workers, although this last group will not affect retired people. All of them are worried about you, but their emotions are affecting you and add more confusion to the already traumatised brain.

Your tendency to try and isolate yourself is affecting others in your environment and there are different reactions and interactions between you and yourself, you and your immediate close family and you and the extended family, as well as your friends.

Stress, anxiety, disruption of relationships, self-pity and depression are some of the emotions that, you. as well as the rest of your world, are going through.

The only thing though that you want from all, yourself included, is to be understood, informed and supported.

Analysing my experience, I mentioned before the relationship with my family members and communication with them was disrupted. I was forced to find a solution on my own, as my doctor was not very helpful. His view was that, as an Orthopaedic Surgeon, I was in a better position than him to find a solution. It could sound logical, but when you are suffering, you need support and possibly communication and reasoning of why you need to do certain things in order to get better. I had none of this.

The solution had to come from me. I spent hours reading and experimenting on myself. All this made me learn a lot, about the parallel reactions we have while we are suffering from chronic pain and believe me, there is a multitude of them. I will try to explain them as simply as I can.

We all know that back pain affects us in a multitude of ways. If we think logically, the original reason that influenced us is the 'damage' of a tissue. This could be a soft tissue (ligament, muscle and disc), or the bone. I am excluding back pain that originates from other organs, like kidneys, pancreas, vessels, etc.

This initial damage creates a localised reaction which, with the help of the nerves, signals the central nervous system (spinal cord and brain), by providing the information. As soon as this information is received, a generalised alert goes through the body and the words 'brace-brace,' similar to when a plane is going to crash-land, is filling our system.

This results in the loss of movement, due to muscle spasm, as the first mechanical reaction. The rigidity of the body, as the brain is forcing muscles to achieve in the attempt to eliminate movement, makes the muscles after time of action,

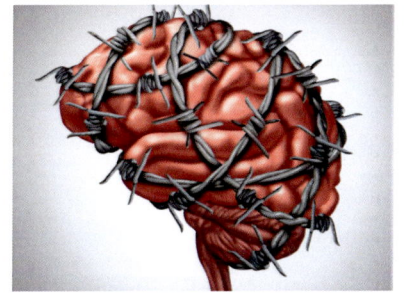

tired. As muscles are overworking, they are asking for more blood supply, necessary to take away the waste they metabolically create with their constant activation. This additional blood supply creates more localised inflammation and swelling, resulting in increased pressure, more pain, more painful signals sent to the brain and more demands for 'brace-brace.'

These demands are given from the area of the hypothalamus in the primary primitive brain and affect the organs (mainly the adrenals, as they produce cortisol, a stress hormone), causing the production of "panic attack" hormones, which in turn affect other organs and finally the pituitary gland. The pituitary gland is located at the base of our brain and is the master gland, communicating all hormonal information to other glands as well as to the cortical brain. This is the initial vicious circle of panic.

I will now try to explain the actions and reactions that I and my loved ones went through during the course of my initial stages of back pain. You may find similarities between your story and mine, which may help you understand the reasons for your reactions at that time.

In my personal case, the following series of effects on myself and my family were observed.

The initial injury has already been described, and there were no neurological findings. I was worried about my condition and wanted answers about the cause of the pain. My doctor investigated me and provided initial treatment in the form of painkillers.

Upon reflecting on my condition, I noticed the different reactions and responses I had demonstrated during the initial stages of my back pain. To facilitate visual understanding, I created the following diagram.

In this first diagram, someone can see how people close to me started to be affected. I was keeping them at a distance, which disrupted our relationship. At the same time, I was focused on my tissue damage problem, and that affected me. It is obvious that initially, my concentration was on the back and the physical characteristics of my pain, but the burden started to shift from the structural physical anatomy to the behavioral elements of myself and my family. During these initial stages, the extended family and friends were not involved. It was a "private" matter.

At the same time, I was experiencing these symptoms, I continued studying and experimenting. However, despite my efforts, there was no improvement. Through my studies, I learned that in cases like mine, when the pain persists and resolves after a period of three months, it is classified as chronic. This is because the brain remains in a state of alert due to hormonal influences, and gradually, a direct relationship between pain and constant struggle begins to form.

HOW BACK PAIN AFFECTS PEOPLE 53

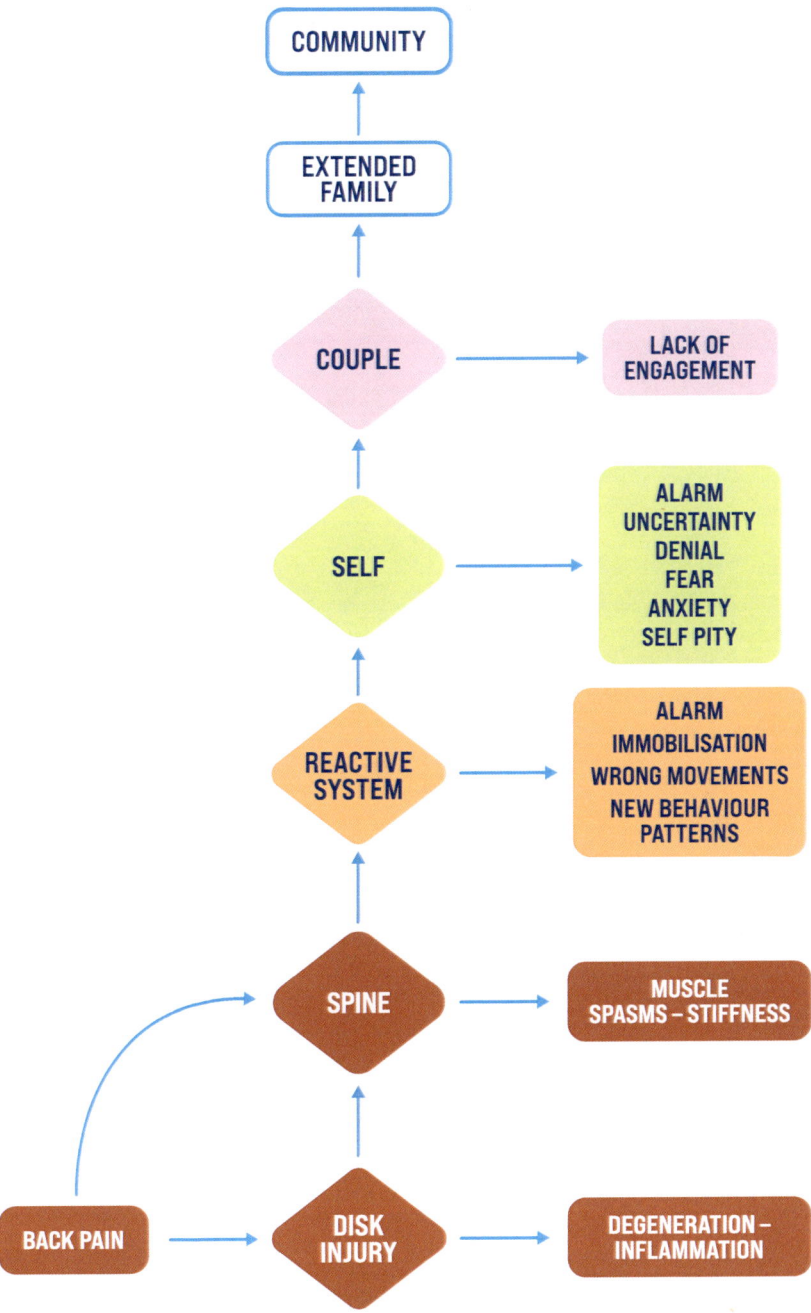

Later on, I will discuss the role of hormones and how they significantly impact our behaviour, as the frontal cortex of our brain is bombarded with panic-inducing information.

Studies have shown that daily mobility is affected, which in turn impacts a person's morale. Uncertainty and anxiety slowly give way to depression, and the combination of immobility and depression negatively affects the sufferer's social life. It is common to hear someone in this situation say, "leave me alone." These changes in social life lead to sleep disorders, problems in family relationships, and so on.

Furthermore, as an individual goes through all these changes, it is discovered that depression, stress, and anxiety have an impact on hormones, leading to additional symptoms such as sleep deprivation. If a lack of social life is added to all these changes, the hormonal imbalance becomes more noticeable, creating an environment for further mental and behavioural disruptive issues.

Both the body and mind enter a state of problem acceptance and spiral downward, exacerbating the pain and depression. This is the vicious cycle of chronic pain, where biology plays a small but constant role, mainly due to the emotional factors that contribute to it.

Unfortunately, the "disruptive" behavioural changes of the sufferer directly affect the close family members, impacting their own hormonal state and causing them to also experience a "panic" condition. Their emotional state becomes strained, creating an emotional domino effect that eventually spreads to the wider community. This situation can lead to a multitude of opinions and confusion.

In the illustration above, it is clear how little space the physical "problems" occupy compared to the combined psychological, social, or behavioural "problems" that are affected by chronic back pain. The physical issues may be the initial presentation, but the rest are the result of various factors and stimuli accumulating over time.

HOW BACK PAIN AFFECTS PEOPLE 55

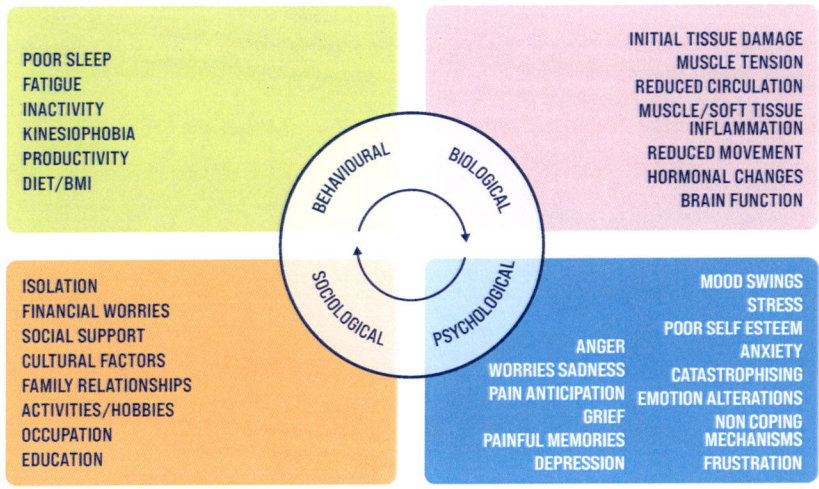

Returning to the observations of my case, since the painkillers did not make a significant difference and I was still in pain, my attitude changed entirely and there was additional stress for everyone involved. The main impact was now evident on the people around me. These emotions were intense, and worries were apparent due to uncertainty about my future outcomes and how my life would progress. My own emotions were not helping them at all. My weight was increasing, and I was concerned and caught in a cycle of self-pity. Blood pressure and stamina were affected.

PAIN MANAGEMENT

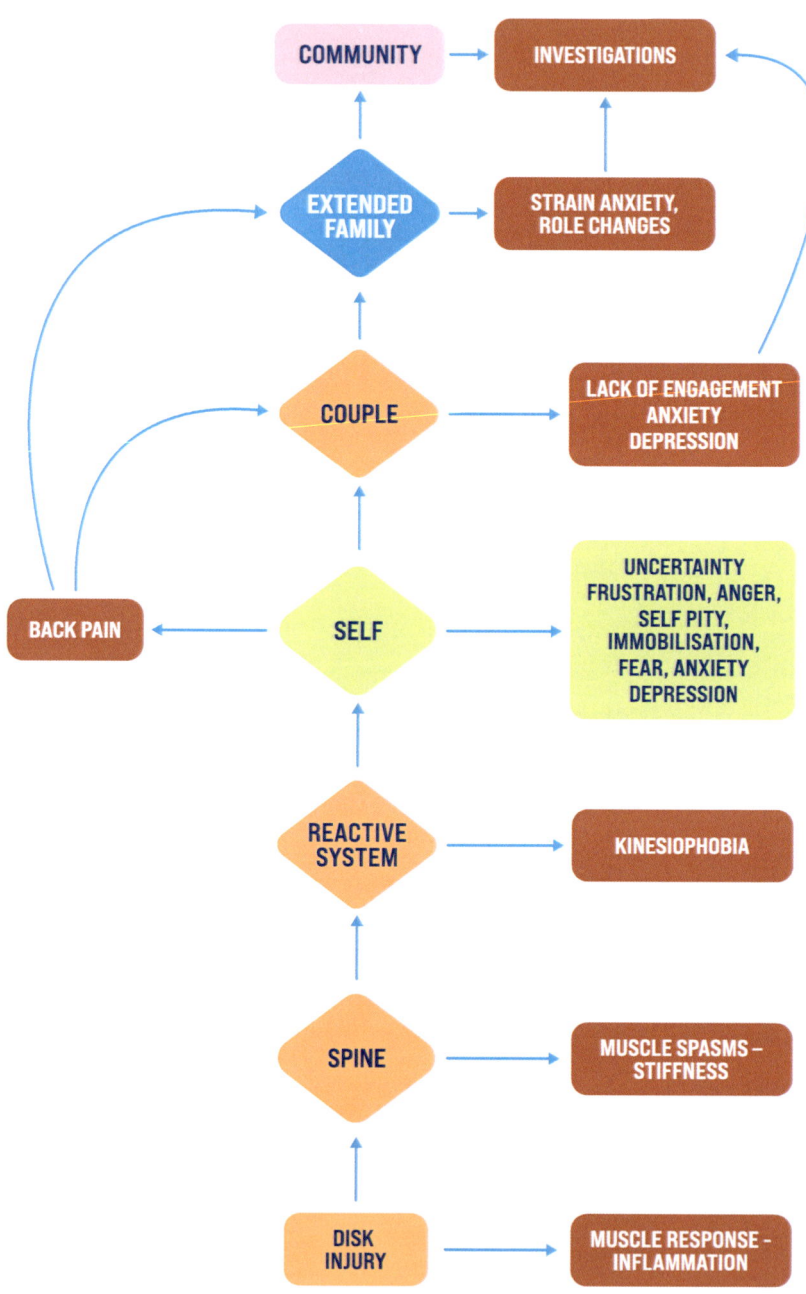

In the diagram above, one can see the changes that were affecting me during this period of my life. I completely ignored my physical pain, and my main concern was constantly reflecting on the facts that resulted from the original injury. I constantly rehearsed the scene of the injury and how it had ruined my activities. I was angry at my doctor and how he managed my needs. I pitied myself and was constantly angry, especially at my colleague who moved at the last minute, wondering what would have happened if he hadn't been there. I was also angry at my doctor's attitude and was not ready to accept the long-standing back pain. I was not a happy person.

The family was under stress, and the extended family was also involved, questioning if it was necessary to involve other physicians or even have further investigations. The potential involvement of the community, friends, or family friends was evident as well.

When my doctor finally announced that I had borderline diabetes and needed constant blood pressure medication, I woke up. My belief that medications and pills had to be eliminated from anyone's thoughts forced me to change. An inner strength began to grow in me. The negative reflections I had been engaging in up until that point transformed into positive thinking, and I started to change. Slowly, I was able to find solutions to my problems.

Once I realised that I was improving, I did what I do best most of the time: further positive reflection. This self-analysis and deep thinking helped me tremendously. I convinced myself that I was cured and my perspective changed completely. Everyone's emotions were reversed, and I mainly focused my thoughts on the original problem, which was the physical/mechanical issue.

This analysis of the different stages of my symptoms led me to a potential diagnosis. As my initial pain and twisted spine improved with another twist, and nothing was evident on the original X-rays, my potential diagnosis was subluxation of the facet joints at some level of my spine. The potential future could involve arthritis of the joints and possible long-term degeneration of the discs.

58 PAIN MANAGEMENT

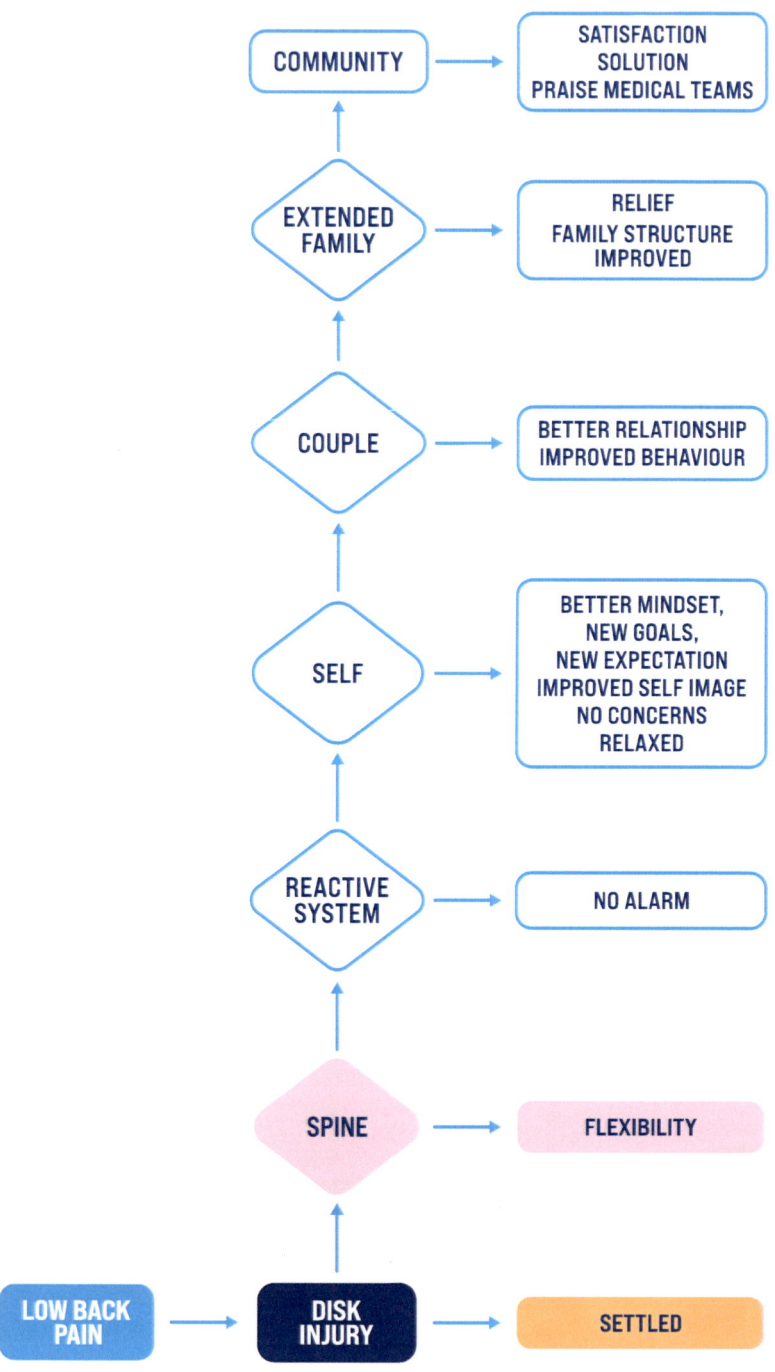

The diagram above shows exactly how the successful "treatment" changed the emotional picture of the family, both extended and close. It also changed the picture of myself and my attitude towards the back pain. It is evident in the positive words that I used.

Based on my story and the changes, one can see that to overcome this labyrinth of physical and emotional trouble, one needs to move in the correct direction slowly and execute each movement step by step. An analysis of the physical/biological part of the circle is necessary. The underlying tissue damage with the rolling effect leads to constant pain.

It is already known that chronic low back pain affects more people on the planet than we can imagine. As age progresses, the incidence of chronic low back pain increases. In the group of people above 65 years old, the most frequent symptoms appear in those who are 80-85 years old, representing 31% of the total. Additionally, 6% of people in this subgroup declare themselves disabled due to their pain symptoms. This is equivalent to 150 million people globally above the age of 80 years old who are disabled because of severe low back pain. They find that these symptoms create a loss of energy and affects them mentally too.

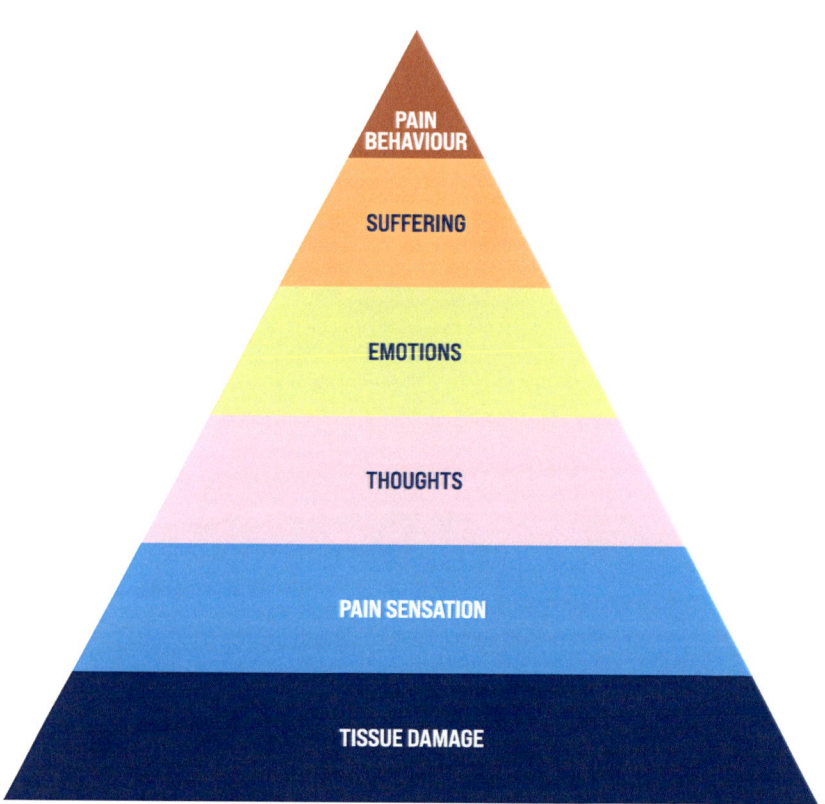

It is obvious from all the diagrams above that the emotional element is greater than any physical issues in a person who is suffering from low back pain. This has a direct effect on the surrounding environment and social circle, affecting the behaviour of a number of people.

This is the vicious circle that you are going through living a life with chronic low back pain, missing the family activities and not being able to enjoy the laughter and company of your grandchildren or not being able to do your hobbies and other daily activities. This is the reason we are here together to walk the journey of symptom management and live a life of better quality.

From my professional experience, I can tell a story of an elderly lady who walked into my consulting rooms. I had seen her in the past and had ordered X-rays. She appeared to have degenerative discs in multiple levels, and she was suffering from osteoporosis (thinning of the bone structure), but she had no obvious compression fracture as a result of it. After she sat in front of me, she mentioned that she feels exhausted due to her constant low back pain.

In her words, she told me that:

"I find that making the bed every morning is a serious business. As I bend over to fix the sheets, I get pain in the back and it takes me forever to get it made. The rest of the housework is torture too. I cannot even do the hoovering or lift the pot from the stove. Standing in front of the sink to wash the dishes is an adventure. I find myself sitting down most of the time or lying down in bed trying to relieve the pain. At night, I cannot sleep well. I am tired at all times. I cannot go anywhere. I lost my friends. My only activity now is opening the fridge and munching on whatever I can find inside it. I feel isolated. Thank God my son arranged once a week for a helper to come over and do the heavy cleaning, but I feel that I am useless. I don't want such a life and I pray to God to take me. I am old, I lived my life. Why do I still live? I don't know. I am debilitated physically, I am an emotional wreck, and I don't know what to do. I am here to ask your opinion if you think that I need to have a trip to Switzerland to organise my voluntary exit from this life. Is it worth spending my few money I put aside?"

Analysis of this grim story and deep analytical thinking can lead to finding out the reasons that pushed this person to say what she said. On physical grounds, she has degeneration and osteoporosis. This is the tissue involvement. This is influencing her psychological sphere as she is worried, has poor self-esteem, she is stressed and catastrophising, she is frustrated and angry with herself, she is sad, and mentally and physically she is expecting the daily pain to be present. Her emotional status is not normal, and she feels that she cannot cope with her condition.

The combination of the physical and emotional elements is affecting her sleep, and as a result, she feels fatigued. Her diet is poor, and although she is not mentioning it, she is gaining weight. Additionally, she is isolated without friends and family, receiving minimal support.

Due to the various issues she is facing, her degree of depression has driven her to make statements of self-destruction.

The question is whether her mental status is affecting her symptoms. It is known from literature that depression and anxiety have an influence on and amplify the symptoms of chronic low back pain. Her physical and mental status collaborate and change due to the constant hormonal influence they have on her central nervous system and the brain's chemistry. Pain itself has become her new existence, as she believes it is the only way she has to live her life. The pain is intertwined with emotions and has become deeply ingrained in her mind, exerting control over her and altering her behaviour.

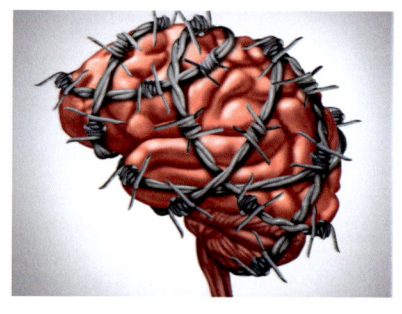

All of the factors mentioned above are influencing her social life, and the absence of it further increases her anxiety. This leads her to continue in a cycle, going around and around. She believes that the only way to break this cycle is to end her life.

"CHEMICAL" EFFECT

It has been demonstrated that patients' chronic pain influences their mechanical and psychological status. They fear that the pain, which is a part of their life, could destroy their future. They are fixated on their pain, constantly expecting to be "hit" by it again and again, which keeps them vigilant. Their anxiety levels are high, and they are constantly stressed. Only negative thoughts are pouring from their mind, and they develop kinesiophobia (fear of movement). They believe that if they move, the pain will come back and the symptoms will worsen. This fear dominates their mind, and their entire being is engulfed in a sea of uncertainty, anger, and desperation.

The situation affects their stress hormones, which in turn affect the primitive part of their brain. Initially, it affects the pituitary gland and ultimately the frontal cortex, where behaviour and emotions are stored. This marks the end of the emotional stage. The emotions are imprinted on the frontal cortex, leading to the formation of new beliefs and habits. Once these are established, they are stored in the cognitive part of the cortex, which serves as the brain's archive. When this information is stored in the brain's archive, it influences the rest of the functional brain. People become prisoners of their own brain, which dictates all bodily functions and thoughts.

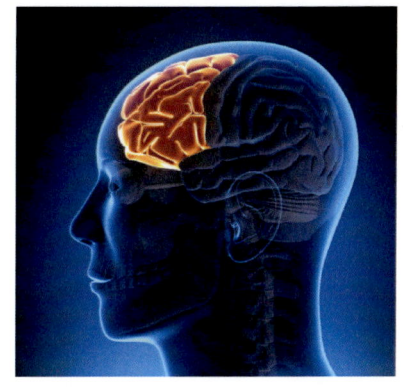

The diagram above shows that the initial stimulus comes to the brown area (primitive brain – Brain stem, Hypothalamus, Amygdala) and via the purple

(Pituitary gland) is influencing the green (Frontal cortex) and then mapped fully in the blue area (Cortical cognitive part) of the brain.

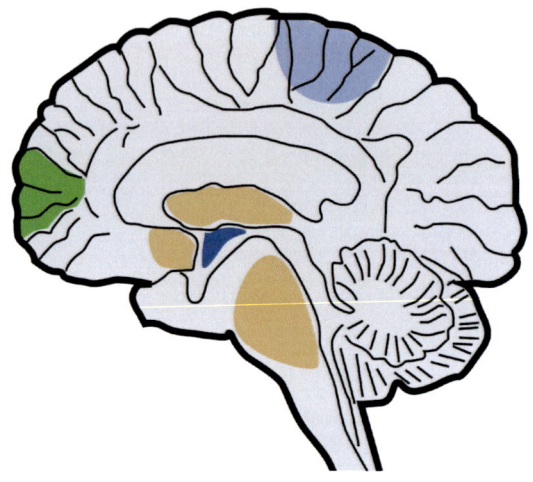

In other words, the majority of us, and I put myself in this group as a chronic low back pain sufferer, are starting to neglect ourselves. Cortisol, one of the stress hormones produced, is constantly bombarding the Hypothalamus and Pituitary Gland, the main central hormone controlling system, which are close to the primitive brain. From there, all the commands fly in the body, resulting in a complete derangement of the rest of the hormones. This way, Thyroxin, Dopamine, and Insulin are affected. The main way of influence is Cortisol, which reduces Dopamine. Dopamine then directly influences Thyroxin by reducing it. The reduced Thyroxin makes us more "relaxed," as it tries to slow down our metabolism, fighting back the effects of Cortisol. This imbalance also creates Insulin resistance, which changes our dietary behaviour, producing the environment for Type 2 diabetes, as it drives us to consume more food. At the same time, it affects the "inflammatory response" of the body. With the activation of this cycle, we eat more, as we try to affect our pleasure hormones, the endorphins, thus it is called comfort eating.

All this activity results in weight gain. Extra weight, as we know, is a mechanical factor that increases the load on your spine. This extra load increases your symptoms of pain and adds more tissue reaction and inflammation. In addition, Insulin is responsible for further tissue inflammation, which can increase our symptoms. Because we are not getting better, our stress levels increase, more Cortisol is produced, and the cycle continues.

DOCTOR'S UNDERSTANDING AND LIMITATIONS

As doctors, we are trained to deal with science. We need hard data, proof, and measurements to carry on with our lives. This is science to you. During our training, we are "asked" to specialise, meaning that we concentrate on a very narrow field where we become experts. However, sometimes we tend to forget the broader picture of the patient's needs.

Hyper-specialisation is great, and there is a need to give expert opinions in difficult cases for the benefit of the patient. But it is necessary to have a panel of doctors from different specialties to achieve this.

Sometimes, we ignore the fact that it is necessary to have a broader knowledge of medicine to allow us to see the person who came for help. A patient needs to be seen as a whole person and not just as a spine, leg, or any other body part. The patient is a human being and needs help in their entirety.

There are times when the Socratic quote "**I know one thing, that I know nothing**" definitely applies to us. We may not know all the answers, and we must be mature enough to inform the patient about it. If necessary, we should say the phrase "I don't know" and ask for help.

But our "ignorance" may be part of our training. The tendency is to treat patients in a reactive, conventional way rather than a preventive or holistic one. We treat pain with painkillers, hypertension (high blood pressure) with hypotensives, and so on. We often prescribe numerous pills to our patients based on the symptoms we see, and if there is even a slight indication, we offer surgery without considering any other solutions to their problems.

During my training, I had the honour to work for about 18 months with a great Spinal Orthopaedic Surgeon. The weekly outpatient clinic had about 45 patients who were suffering from back pain at different stages, some at the beginning of their journey and some already operated on or presenting problems months after their surgery. In our discussions, this mentor of mine said that we should only offer an operation to 4% of the patients presenting with back pain, even if they had neurological findings. The reason is that often these symptoms improve on their own.

So the offered treatments were mainly non-operative, and if there was a need for an operation, it was only offered to people with neurological pressure that was not improving with any other means. It was made clear to them that the procedure is meant to relieve the pain that radiates to the leg and that they may have permanent back pain for the rest of their lives due to surgical scarring. I was "cruelly" saying all this to the patients before their surgery as part of the informed consent. But, as everyone can see, my training was based on mechanical/physical solutions.

During all the training years, I was not told anything about hormones' involvement with pain or how they influence the brain and change our body functions and behaviour, including our psychology. I had to experience it myself and be forced to go back to books to find ways to improve physical, hormonal, and mental issues.

💡 ACTIVITY

Focus on the physical and mental reactions you had, after you saw your physician and the treatment you went through.

How are you affected by your symptoms?

Concentrate on mental and emotional recovery by either exercising or engaging in mindfulness practice in order to give your prefrontal cortex a break from chaotic thoughts and emotions.

SOLUTION PLANNING: 5 P'S CREATING THE 5 M'S STRATEGY

What do you think a person who has been a back pain sufferer needs to be provided so that they would be able to manage the symptoms better?

Do you think that investigations, information, or an operation would be the answer?

On the other hand, is a better understanding of the cause and reason of the symptoms a better solution?

Do you think that a permanent solution could be the answer?

Does a permanent cure or elimination of the symptoms exist?

The real answer to these questions is complex. You will need more information, and this would be obtained through the correct examination and investigations if necessary. This way, the reason would be obvious, and as soon as the cause is known, possibly the solution may be clearer. On the other hand, if someone is searching for a permanent solution to eliminate the symptoms, they are living in a utopian land. From the moment back pain knocks on your door and appears in your body, and if the symptoms develop to become chronic, the word "elimination" must not exist in your vocabulary.

Now, by reading this cruel statement above, you may become more depressed and go hide in your dark corner. Your brain will be further alarmed as you were just told that the pain will be there at all times. Don't be disheartened, as the word "elimination" could be replaced by the word "management." I can assure you that the pain will not be there at every moment of your life. The best way to describe it is that pain has the ability to visit you sometimes, but you will be given the armamentarium to fight it back and stay on top of it. Think that you have the ability to turn the volume down, and it is up to you to learn how much pain you will allow your body to have.

Back pain symptoms can be managed in a way that their presence will be so infrequent that you may think that you have eliminated back pain.

This is the reason why we are here: to discuss and find out together the systematic plan mapping which will give the solution to back pain symptoms. I am here to help you and share my experiences and teach you ways to manage and improve your symptoms.

You already know, as it has been mentioned, about my back injury in the operating theatre and how my doctor never gave me the necessary attention, as he was telling me:

"You are an Orthopaedic Surgeon and you know what to do."

As a patient, though, I needed support and information; information that possibly I could have if I could undergo any further investigations. Unfortunately, I was not and I am not allowed to self-refer for any investigations, due to existing policies. Everything has to be suggested and agreed upon by my doctor, who had no interest in sending me for any imaging other than a simple X-ray, which reported that I had no congenital spinal deformities and no fractures. I already knew that, and for me, it was irrelevant.

1. What else was wrong? His belief was that all the symptoms were due to muscular problems, which I could not disagree with, but he decided to only prescribe throat pills. At the same time, he was not referring me to physiotherapy, stating that "all this will improve on its own."

    The alternate option I had and was able to pursue was finding a solution myself. I started my research and was determined to improve.

To do that, I had to delve deep and try to understand the cause of my symptoms and find a solution once I understood it. But how could I find the cause without being able to see data, meaning investigations?

I concluded that I needed to reflect and concentrate on the solution, and try to find the way to my improvement. To achieve this, I created segments of the main fields I had to tackle. These segments eventually produced the 5 P's.

1. Power
2. Purpose
3. Passion
4. Plan
5. Productivity

Anyone would think that this is a finely tuned philosophy, and possibly this is what happens to someone when they concentrate on the depth of their soul. Others look at them as if they're from Mars.

But I ignore all these thoughts and present to you my initial guides for my journey out of my misery.

This is only part of my solution, but what does each P represent?

The first is the body's muscle **power**. It represents a healthy being that is not afraid to move. A body that can be used for daily activities and thrive. A body that is given to us by our Creator, and is something we need to cherish. There is an ancient Greek quote by Aristotle, "A healthy mind in a healthy body." This tells us that if we look after our bodies, we are also looking after our minds, as these two interact. To create a healthy body, we need to:

- Keep moving and exercise.
- Look after the fuel you put in your body. Nutrition is the key. Nutrients are not only the physical food that you digest, but also the thoughts you feed your brain too.

- Plan for the above and stay committed - if you think that you are having trouble sticking to the plan, have another person who will be able to help you, like a trainer or a member of your family to keep an eye on your progress.

The more you get in shape, the more confidence you will have, and your brain gets more active and content. Confidence gives you a feeling of self-assurance, reduces feelings like fear, self-doubt and removes any worrying thoughts. When you are confident, you are feeling and eventually getting more motivated too.

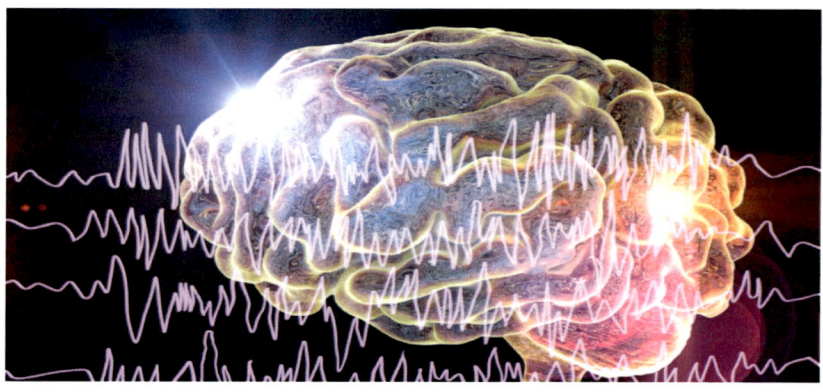

As Dr Daniel Amen, renounced Neuropsychologist, stated: **"Remove ANTs (Autonomous Negative Thoughts) from your brain as they may eat it."**

Protect your brain from these thoughts.

It is necessary to fix someone's thoughts and protect them. You have to develop a meaning, a goal you need to focus on and fight to reach it, using positive attitudes and thoughts. To achieve it, you develop a **purpose**.

Protecting your mind and wellbeing is your purpose, so you need to be dedicated to look after your powerful and beautiful thoughts that you have. Compare your mind to a big farm - you are the farmer.

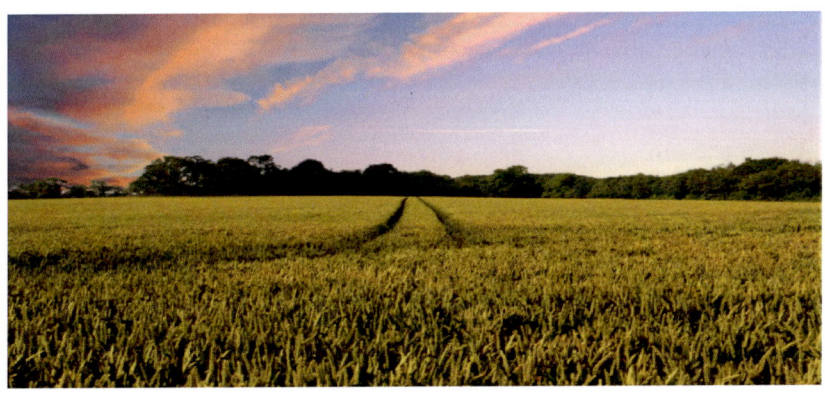

Whatever seeds you will plant, determine the kind of crop you will produce. So, you need to plant high-quality seeds that will yield fruitful plants and not weeds. Your mind is like a power plant that facilitates your decision-making. You cannot control every thought that pops into your mind, just as a farmer cannot control which seeds will be carried by the wind onto their farmland. However, you can control how you react to these thoughts and decide whether to act upon them or ignore them. Just as a farmer may allow a small daisy to flourish at the edge of their field, they will remove any weeds that are spreading within the crop.

In order to have a happy and healthy mind, you should start your day with positive thoughts and establish a routine that supports this process. It is similar to how a farmer would come early in the morning to 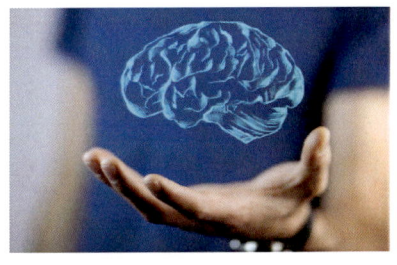 water their field. Avoid starting your day with worrying negative thoughts, and instead focus on feelings of joy and gratitude. It is the beginning of a new day, and the sun is shining brightly in the sky. The *next thing* to be done was to fix the relationships. As you achieve more by looking after your body and mind, you will start to become

passionate and get easily connected with your environment. You will also develop better and stronger relationships with the people who are around you. You have to keep the loved ones close and allow them to assist you in your journey. **Exercise** can help your brain release endorphins, hormones responsible for your happiness.

This way, you are "falling in love" with your surroundings. Being with people you love and appreciate for the help they provide to you can also release endorphins. By giving them back the gratitude they deserve, the circle of happiness is complete. On the other hand, you become so powerful, passionate, and protective of your well-being that people who create feelings of anger, sadness, anxiety, depression, and other negative thoughts are removed from your life. It is understood that you cannot have great control over others, but you can control yourselves. Therefore, by the power of your mind, you can eliminate toxic, negative environments around you.

You need to be aware of your actions, so you need to **plan** ahead. You need to prearrange the kind of music you will listen to, the book you will read and every task you need to fulfil your goals. It is advisable to plan your daily activities before you go to bed, so you don't have to worry about them in the morning. This way you remove the chances of anxiety and any negative thoughts.

You need to find ways to balance work and personal life. The majority of people make the mistake to concentrate on their jobs and forget about their family. This way, they lose contact, and they are unilaterally passionate. This creates confusion to you. It is good to focus on **productivity** but you must be balanced. Your environment has to be balanced. You have to be balanced. You have to be productive, but at the same time, organised. Productivity-centred on one person alone could indicate a lack of confidence, leading to the need to constantly check everything around. This lack of confidence can create anxiety and stress. You must work together with your loved ones and trust each other. If you want to be trusted, you must learn to trust others. By working in a community with a common purpose, you become more successful. If you feel that your product is not good enough and needs improvements, you can rely on your co-workers and ask for help. If there is still a problem, you can bring in a more experienced person to assist. Becoming productive in a correct and positive way boosts your confidence and creates a better future overall.

But you may wonder how these 5 P's help with your back pain.

The explanation is simple.

Move and exercise to take care of your body. Commit to a program with passion. Spend time with and appreciate your loved ones and friends. Set goals and have a purpose for a better future by taking care of your mind. Plan future actions in an organised way that can help you achieve your goals, and don't hesitate to ask others for assistance.

To make this happen you need to start by planning your day and move one step at the time. You have to start by:

- Becoming an early riser.
- Think about everyday's outcome in a positive way.
- Remove the 'ANTs' from your brain.
- Listen to music, read a book and meditate.
- Take care of the body, as the body is a temple, by eating and drinking the correct food; drink a lot of water.
- Exercise daily and create a habit of it.
- Appreciate life and smile throughout the day.
- Think positively.
- Embrace the Epicurean quote "*What is good is easy to get and what is terrible is easy to endure,*" meaning that a smile or a nice word (the good), is easy to receive or give and every challenge is an opportunity to win. Don't complain!

After I injured my back in the operating theatre and analysed my feelings, I found myself alone. This was not anybody else's fault except my own. As a result, I gained weight, my blood pressure went through the roof, and I 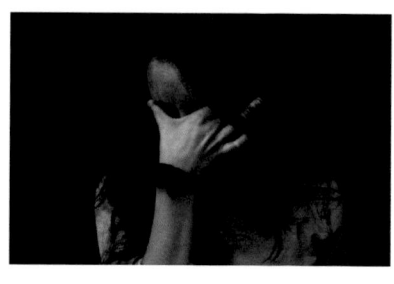 became breathless even when attempting to climb a flight of stairs. My family doctor classified me as obese and borderline diabetic, and the only treatment offered to me was more "chemistry." Like all doctors, my doctor believed in pills and was giving me handfuls of them. He started with painkillers, which I understood for the acute initial phase, but he continued trying to "treat the rest of my pathological symptoms" such as blood pressure and blood sugar.

Personally, I don't like pills and I don't know anybody who likes them. My defense mechanism against my doctor's advice was to ask for time to think about it. He gave me an ultimatum of six months, so I went back to my favorite subject, second to operating: research. I was accepting the painkillers at the moment, but I was concentrating on finding ways to avoid taking any more.

I studied anatomy again, as well as the physiology of movement and chronic pain, biomechanics of the spine, endocrinology, and the effects of pain on the body and mental well-being. I also delved into some uncomfortable internal medicine in an effort to find solutions. Finally, I created a plan.

I experimented on myself and created statistics based on my own body observations. I was determined to avoid any more pills except for the light painkillers.

By following and analysing the 5 P's and after a lot of trial and error experimentation, I developed the 5 M's strategy:

I called it the '5 M's Strategy,' and it is as follows:

1. Motion
2. Music
3. Mental awareness
4. Meditation
5. Marking down

During that time, as I went through the different stages of this strategy, I had a patient come for consultation. She was a 67-year-old woman complaining of low back pain. Her symptoms began about 20 years ago when she slipped and fell on ice in a sitting position on a winter morning. She was examined and investigated at that time, and the given diagnosis was "soft tissue injury of the back." She was sent for physiotherapy. Her initial symptoms improved over time, but she was left with chronic dull pain at the bottom of her spine that frequently changed to more severe pain, which she referred to as 'crisis.' When she came to me, she was in this state of crisis and she had very limited spinal movement, a stiff back, and pain that radiated throughout her back from her shoulder blades down to her buttocks. She was afraid to even make minimal movements. Her radiological investigations, including plain X-rays and an MRI, confirmed moderate to severe degeneration, with obvious arthritic changes in the bones and dehydrated discs.

There was no nerve compression. She asked for strong painkillers and declined physiotherapy due to her fear of movement. Further discussion revealed that she had lost almost all of her friends because she preferred to stay at home. Her only source of entertainment was her TV, and she constantly snacked. Her BMI was high, as she had gained about 25 kilos (55 pounds) in the past few months. She didn't even want to step on a scale and refused to do so during our consultation because she was ashamed of her body.

She reminded me a lot of myself. So, I decided to talk to her about the different treatment options she had, without relying on strong painkillers, and how we could alleviate her pain and make slow progress towards a better future. I told her that she would have to work for this and assured her that I was confident she would achieve very good results. I was cautious in initially mentioning movement and music, and I lightly touched on the topic of meditation and journaling, as she was sensitive about it. However, I did discuss the importance of mental awareness, emphasising that she needed to forget about how her pain started and focus on her future goals. I explained to her that my recommendations were based solely on my own observations and had not been scientifically proven in published papers.

She left the consultation room with questions in her mind, but also with enthusiasm to implement this new method of treatment.

A few months later, I saw her again and she mentioned that she had lost weight and experienced improvement in her pain. She had fewer crisis moments and felt happier. She had also reduced her use of painkillers and was confident that she would continue to improve in the future.

I wasn't sure if this was something worth pursuing further or if it was just a coincidence. That's the scientific mindset, after all.

Once again, I tried to keep everything to myself, delving deeper and analysing further. I even started experimenting on myself. Eventually, I made the decision to document my proposed pathway based on the scientific analysis I had conducted.

> **I ONCE MORE SAY THAT THE WHOLE CONCEPT IS BASED ON MY OWN OBSERVATIONS AND STUDIES, AND IT IS NOT REPLACING ANY MEDICAL CONSULTATION OR OPINION OF THE INDIVIDUAL PHYSICIAN THAT IS LOOKING AFTER YOU. IT IS SERVING ONLY AS EDUCATIONAL PURPOSES.**

So let's start to analyse this strategy together by dissecting into its different segments.

MOTION

The first thing the brain does in a state of emergency is to order immobilisation. The condition of kinesiophobia (fear of motion) is developed. This order given from the brain to the rest of the body is led by fear, as you remember in the case of my lady patient. You need to fight this. It is known that movement or better exercises can make you happy, as the brain releases endorphins. The easiest way to treat this is to start short walks. The initial walk could be around the own yard, around the block, or a stroll down to do some window shopping. One or two times around the block may be enough to start, but the number can increase as time goes by. The frequency can be once or twice per week in the initial stages, but gradually it can become a daily routine.

As the energy levels increase, the distance can increase and slowly some exercises may be added. These exercises can be the initial stretching and rotational movements of the torso but can slowly increase in complexity and frequency.

Increased movement gives you the confidence that motion is not bad, and this way you treat your kinesiophobia. If there is an opportunity to join a gym or do exercises in water, like aqua aerobics or swimming, it would be very beneficial. Don't forget that when you are in water, gravity and thus the load on the joints are lesser. So, water is very beneficial.

The exercises have to take in consideration the function of the different groups of muscles and the direction of their fibres. You need to activate and strengthen the dorsal and abdominal muscles as well as improve the flexibility of the iliopsoas muscle, the muscle that links the spine to the hip. You need to remember that creating a six-pack abdomen is not the only solution, as the rest of the abdominal muscles at the sides of the body have a different fibre orientation than the frontal muscles, so we need a combination of exercises.

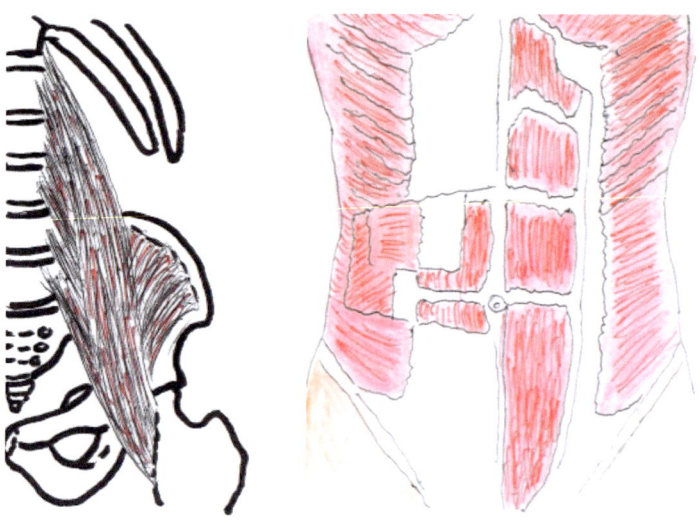

In the diagrams, it is obvious that the iliopsoas muscle is present. However, also concentrate on the direction of the muscle fibres at the different levels of the abdominal muscles. Only the rectus abdominis (the 6-pack muscle) has a direction from top to bottom. The rest of the abdominal and core muscle fibres have either oblique or transverse (horizontal) directions. Notice that different exercises are necessary for these muscles.

Motion is the key factor in our attempt to stimulate our brain and overcome the fear of movement.

MUSIC – MOVIES

It is evident that art has a clear influence on our emotions. The most well-studied art form is music, followed by movies as they combine visual and acoustic stimuli. Music combines rhythm, harmony, pitch, melody, and meter.

Pythagoras, the Greek philosopher, was the first to take a scientific approach towards music and studied the ways in which it influences us. He described in mathematical terms how musical notes or compositions can be either pleasant or unpleasant to our ears. He found that music with a regular sequence and lower pitch is more pleasant, as it produces more harmonious waves and is also easier to understand mathematically.

Music is one of the means that has made us happy, relaxed, and mobile since our young age. Our mothers know this well. It is a form of stimuli that influences our brain, particularly in the emotional sphere.

You have favourite tracks that make you move and dance quietly, even when you are alone, as soon as you hear them. There are other tracks that make you stay silent and delve deep into your thoughts, and those that may help you fall asleep.

Let's not forget that in the beginning of our lives, our mothers sang lullabies to help us fall asleep.

Music influences your brain in more than one area. It affects both the ancient and secondary parts of your brain. The areas involved are the insula (yellow), hypothalamus (red), amygdala (dark blue), and pre-frontal cortex (brown).

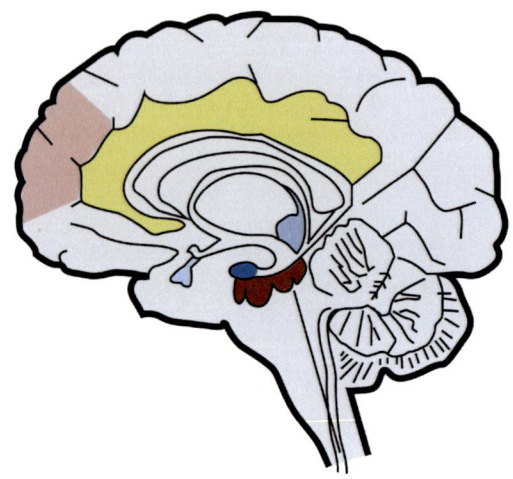

The hypothalamus and amygdala are part of the ancient brain. The hypothalamus controls body temperature, hunger, thirst, and mood, and it directly influences the pituitary gland (shown in light blue), which in turn influences all the other glands.

Through the release of hormones, your metabolism can be changed, as well as the frequency of your pulse, appetite, awareness, and behaviour. These hormonal changes and their effects on your functions are directly linked to the circles, loops, and logical sequence of the waves created by the rhythm, tone, acceleration, and intensity of music.

The main hormones produced are oxytocin, arginine-vasopressin, and endorphins, primarily produced in the hypothalamus and pituitary gland, and dopamine, produced in the adrenals. Dopamine is responsible for a person's good mood. All these hormones directly influence our emotions, as well as other hormones, and can alter our metabolic state.

Both oxytocin and dopamine suppress cortisol (also produced by the adrenals), reducing anger, stress, anxiety, and depression. Arginine-vasopressin influences and reduces the cardiac rhythm and blood pressure. Dopamine can also affect thyroxin (a hormone involved in activity and alertness) and insulin (a hormone that controls blood sugar) by reducing their levels. On the other hand, testosterone (an androgenic hormone that also impacts activity and alertness) increases. Testosterone has been found to control pain.

Listening to soft, easy listening music or gentle classical music has been found to increase oxytocin, endorphins, arginine-vasopressin, dopamine, testosterone, while decreasing thyroxin and insulin. This can help us to calm down and improve our mood, making us more positive about our future.

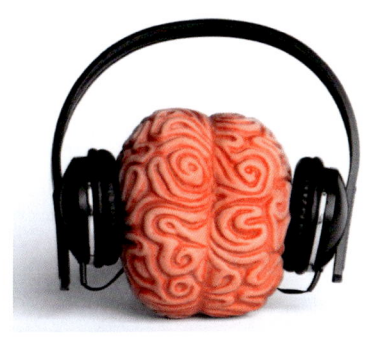

On the other hand, hard rock, punk music, and certain classical compositions, such as those by Wagner, have the opposite effect on us, putting us in a state of alertness. This is why soft music would not be very helpful when driving long distances, although it can be beneficial in traffic jams as it helps to lower our stress levels. Some researchers also blame rock music for physical trauma that can be caused by repetitive movements of our spine, which can worsen our symptoms.

In the elderly population, researchers claim that easy listening music alleviates the psychological states of anxiety, tension, and stress in individuals.

Based on all of the above, we can consider music as an alternative "medication" to decrease the factors that amplify the symptoms of those suffering from chronic low back pain.

Similar effects are observed with the type of movies we watch. Researchers conducted an experiment by dividing a group of individuals into three sub-groups. The first group had to watch romantic

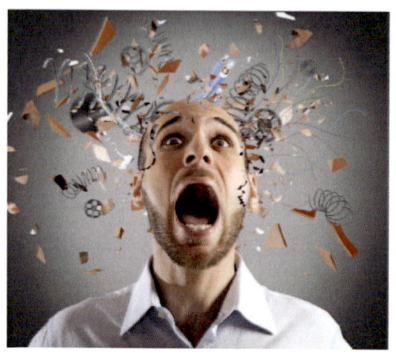

family films or comedies, the second group watched action and horror films, and the third group watched documentaries. The hormones of all individuals were measured before and after the film. They found that the first group had low stress hormones and were calmer, having a similar effect to people who listen to easy listening music. The second group had elevated stress hormones, and the third group had no difference between their two readings.

In summary, it is better for you to listen to easy listening music and soft classics, or watch romantic films and comedies, as they help reduce our stress levels and anxiety. It is necessary to avoid Punk Rock and Horror films if the goal is to become calmer.

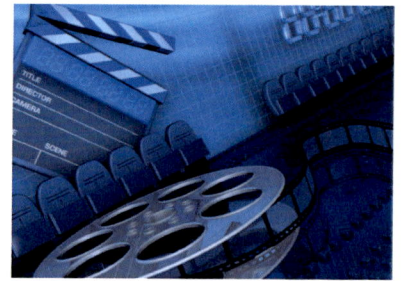

Therefore, music is a practice that can be used for your benefit to escape from your "misery."

MEDITATION

This can be a combination of music and movement, or it could even involve the lack of it. The purpose is to help the mind focus and concentrate on positive thoughts and goals that everyone has. I can tell you that by taking a trip to favourite places, you may find help and become calmer. Being calm, you will be able to follow practices that can help you stay focused on a specific task and train your mind to have a positive outcome.

You can practice this in a quiet room or by listening to music indoors or outdoors. Some people prefer to be in specific spots in nature or concentrate by doing specific exercises, like yoga.

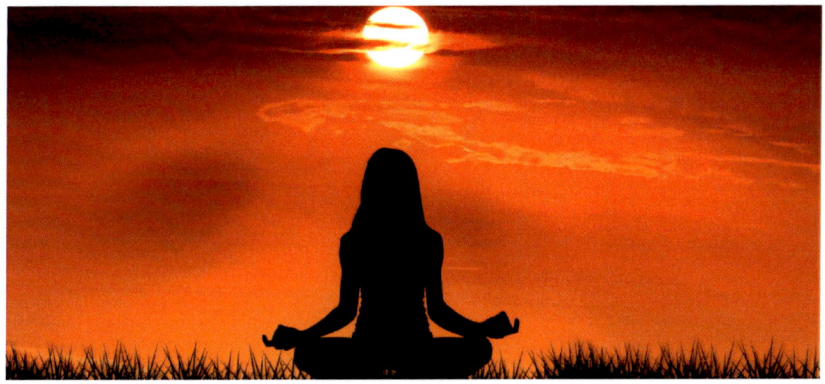

To have this desired positive effect, someone has to develop a strong belief in an idea or a desired outcome and react in a positive way in an attempt to remove any existing obstacles. Concentration on the present goal and visualisation of it, assisted by controlling your physical reactions at the same time, is necessary. Strong focus on the purpose, in the present moment without judgement or fear about anything you may find in your future life. Deep concentration within the mind itself is necessary to be achieved, using all mental and physical power to focus on that specific belief and feel in your mind that it is happening.

As mentioned, in most cases, the use of soft music or a tranquil environment can help concentration.

MENTAL AWARENESS

This is a constant process for the refinement of our goals; it is not one of progress. It is something you have to repeat frequently as your circumstances change. You have to use it to clarify yourself and plan your actions. This way, you will avoid any distractions from your environment or even from your own self.

There are some steps you have to take:

1. *Reflection*: You need to be able to analyse the state you are in at present, pinpoint it and find out what is influencing it.
2. *Love yourself*: Be kind and calm with your emotions and feelings. Imagine the life you want, and you are dreaming to have and embrace it. Plan for it and live for this future 'ideal but realistic' life. Fill your mind with happy emotions. If you find yourself in a dark place, you may start feeling numb and stay there simply because you are "living in the moment", trapping yourself within it and becoming unable to escape. Avoid dwelling on painful memories or fearing any kind of change. *The majority of our fears are not real or useful.* Become a positive person.
3. *Control*: Become disciplined and persist on the goals you have set out to achieve. Be able to control yourself. *"A man who cannot control self is not free"* – Pythagoras. So become free.
4. *Flow*: Become able to create a path so well defined that the actions and thoughts will flow freely, as water flows from the river to the sea.
5. *Willingness* to improve self: To achieve it, you need to think with such intensity about the ideal future destination and believe in this new change you are planning for your life. Love this change, become enthused of this change, dream of this and be happy of being changed. Do not look back to the

dark life. Create a strong will to improve your life, one step at the time and continue progressing.

Following all of the above, you must plan, work hard, and stay on the path. You need to start by assessing your current condition, and this needs to be acknowledged.

You must acknowledge that back pain is real and a fact. It takes time to comprehend and accept that back pain is a persistent issue, and the only thing you can do is confront it and enhance the quality of your life without fear.

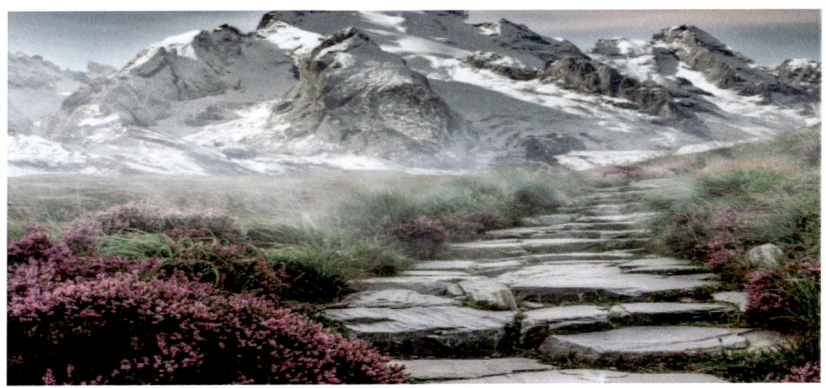

Depression and anxiety caused by any physical problems are acknowledged and accepted.

The future objective is envisioned. The path you need to take in order to reach your goal must be contemplated and planned.

The path is nicely paved with slabs and you have to walk on them, stepping on them one step at a time. Follow this path, focusing on your purpose. The direction has to be clear and focused on the goal. Reverse engineering can also be used to help you achieve your arrival at your destination. Imagine that you have already been to your desired spot. Then turn back and see the path you have walked, and you can track all the steps you need to take on your way to your future goal.

You know that you need to follow this road step by step and one step at a time, and only this way will you reach your ideal outcome. The need to analyse the reasons you have that drive you to this change is paramount. You need to know why you need to change. Then you need to answer what you have to do to achieve the change and, in turn, achieve your goal.

The thought that is planted in your mind has to be so intense that it will create a new behaviour pattern, like the groove water can create on the rock. The deeper the groove, the more efficient it is, and it is easy to be filled with more water, facilitating the flow of it to the river and ultimately to the final destination. The more frequent and more intense the thought is, the deeper the "groove."

Your goal is to strengthen all your new thoughts with repetition and perseverance, and in this way, you are supporting your behavioural change.

You must not be afraid if there are times when you find yourself in a situation that is not the preferred one. You are not a loser. Create this mental picture: When you want to learn how to dance, you go to a dancing instructor and ask them to teach you the moves. When you learn them, you are asked to go to the fair and dance in front of all the people. It will be normal to step on some toes or even lose the steps or the rhythm, but you persevere and insist on dancing. This way, you start becoming an expert.

There are people who say that they don't need an expert to show them the ways to improve. Is this a sound attitude? If you want to play the guitar and you don't go to an instructor, then the only thing you learn to do is make noise. You must remember that if you don't want to be instructed by an expert in the field, you may have a potential issue with criticism.

Aristotle was preaching that to have a well-developed mental awareness you need to firstly recognise your own feelings and be able to manage them, and secondly you need to be able to recognise the feelings of your fellow humans and be flexible, not to offend them.

By saying this, you have to become able to understand yourself, find your goal, your destiny, and make sure that you know why you want to be there, plan your way, start your journey by finding how you will do it. If you are not clear how to do it, make an anagram of the *HOW and replace it with the word WHO*, as Tony Robbins says. There is always someone who has made the journey, and he/she will help you manage it with their help if necessary, and they may help you be accountable for your actions.

This is my role. I am here to assist you and share my experiences; this way you will thrive to a better quality of life by managing your back pain better.

Planning, repetition, and perseverance are helping you develop confidence and motivation for your future achievements. All of these also influence, on the other hand, your hormonal balance.

Hormones and emotions interact, as was explained, meaning that the frontal cortex has new imprints and thus creates new habits. In other words, you need to get into a state of happiness. I am not implying the use of "chemistry" for that, as I am against any medicinal help.

It is found that achieving happiness is not a passive path; rather, you need to take action. Real happiness is not connected to material possessions. It is something that you live and experience. Certain activities have been found to easily lead to happiness. Typically, you need to be focused on something that is very interesting to you and fully engages your mind. You need to have fun during these activities. You need to enjoy what you do, and in doing so, you contribute to your spiritual well-being.

Engaging in pleasurable activities, such as social gatherings or creative pursuits, can increase your confidence. Increased confidence leads to greater enthusiasm and motivation. Being enthusiastic and motivated generates feelings of happiness, which in turn stimulates your frontal cortex. This positive influence on your overall behaviour promotes a more optimistic outlook. This change can also impact the pituitary gland and your entire hormonal system. It is well-known that physical activity leaves a person feeling content, relaxed, and with a positive attitude, as it triggers the release of endorphins throughout the body.

It is important to find ways to engage both your mind and body, while also having a clear dream that you wish to achieve. Remember that the treasure you seek exists within yourself and not elsewhere. Follow the guidance of Dr. Daniel Amen, a renowned neuro-psychologist with international recognition, who advises destroying the ANTs (Autonomous Negative Thoughts) that poison your brain and diminish your treasure. Love and protect your brain.

When reviewing the aforementioned subjects as the starting point, destination, rationale, and means to achieve your goals and bring about change, ensure that you question and answer them within yourself. Protect your brain and your thoughts.

In other words, these are the questions you need to answer:

- Where are you?
- Where do you want to go?
- Why do you need to do this?
- What do you have to do to achieve change?
- How will you do it?

Answering these questions will help you establish your current status, visualise your future goals, find the reasons that are pushing you to change, and discover ways to make them happen.

MARKING DOWN

Chronic pain, as already mentioned, can drive you to anxiety and depression. This is the result of your own worries, in addition to hormonal imbalance. This hormonal derangement starts with the influence of cortisol on thyroxin and insulin, via the stimulation of the brain and the main endocrine glands within it, and the effect these have on our behaviour.

One of the common reactions of a depressed person's attitude is a huge dive into the fridge. In other words, to achieve a change in your newly developed dietary habits, you need to retrain your brain in a way that it will be 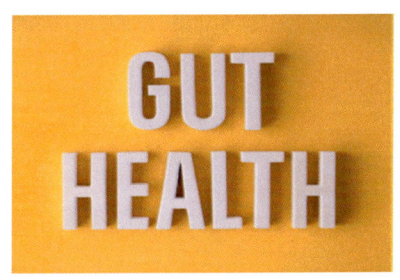 accepted as the new norm, and it will become a permanent habit. The need for you to create these new habits and beliefs is fundamental if you want to correct the outcome.

The main goal is for you to create a permanent solution, and to do so, you need to transform yourself. You need to establish new habits that can lead you to successful weight loss.

On the other hand, you have to remember that weight loss is only a numbers game. If you don't undergo a deep-rooted transformation, staying on the surface of just counting numbers, you will ultimately end up losing. The reason for this failure is the lack of a solid foundation for permanent change. In other words, you must train your brain if you want to achieve this.

An additional reason for this behaviour is the "secondary brain" you have in your gut. It is known that in your digestive system, there are approximately 40 trillion bacteria of different species living in harmony, and they are called the microbiome.

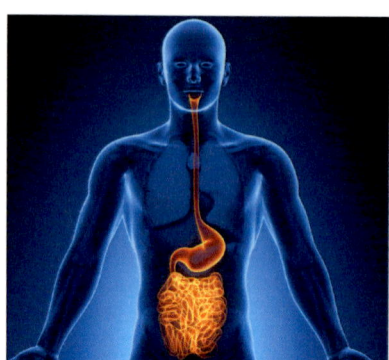

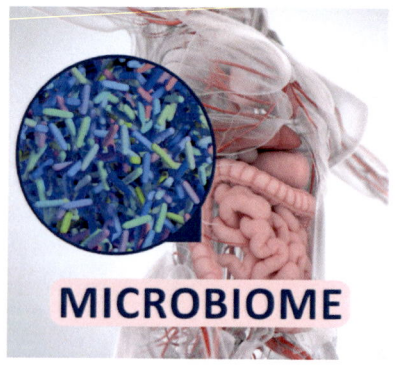

MICROBIOME

They are very important for your health, and they can be influenced by the food you consume. The wrong type of foods can upset them and may cause them to react in a way that creates "unhappy" conditions for you. These bacteria are capable of producing substances that can influence your hormones, or they can produce specific hormones themselves.

If a certain species of bacteria becomes dominant, they can overpower the rest of the species and demand only to be fed and thrive. They can demand a particular type of food because they like it more. In other words, these bacteria can easily dictate your appetite and force you to eat whatever they want.

On the contrary, if there is a balance, all the species are happy, and your appetite is balanced. This way, your diet is balanced.

A separate factor that can influence your weight control is stimulation of **autophagy**.

What is autophagy? It is the ability of your body cells to repair themselves. It is a biological automatic maintenance work your cells do constantly. As soon as they find out that something within them is malfunctioning, they have the ability to destroy it by consuming it in their attempt to function more efficiently. As cells grow older, they accumulate "bad" proteins within their plasma. These can make their "life" difficult, and their response to the problem is repair by destruction.

The term "autophagy" derives from two Greek words: "auto" = "self" and "phagein" = "eating," in other words, cells eat themselves.

This ability that the cells have can make the body function better and help you lose weight.

Can you stimulate autophagy? The answer is YES.

The main factor that can initiate it is fasting, and if exercising is added, autophagy is amplified.

Are there any other factors that can stimulate autophagy? Exercise is mentioned, and vigorous exercise is found to be better, although daily activities or daily exercise of different levels of intensity are sufficient enough to stimulate it.

Except for fasting and exercising, there are some foods that can stimulate autophagy, although the results are based only on laboratory experiments and not on live humans.

Do you need to be afraid of fasting? Do you think that you will be deprived of any nutrients during that period?

It is known to all that people over the centuries did not have the ability of food abundance. In the years when Neanderthals were living, people were hunting for their food. There was a combination of exercising and uncertainty of finally finding food. This meant that they may have had fasting periods until the next kill. But they were not weak people. They could function to their full potential.

Later on, several religions implemented fasting periods within their ceremonial calendar. It is a common practice to omit food under certain circumstances, so do not fear fasting.

There are many different schemes and diets based on fasting patterns.

These are based on long fasting periods of religious functions, but also there are others based on intermittent fasting during different time periods, such as the day or the week. Within a week, you can miss a couple of days, the 2:5 scheme, or if the chosen time period is a day, the 16:8 (16 hours fasting and 8 hours that you can eat) scheme is applied.

During fasting time, people can drink water or consume elements that keep the microbiome happy.

So to keep them healthy and "happy," you need to take care of them.

There are people who do not accept that intermittent fasting can influence weight loss and insist on calorie calculations.

Calorie calculation, though, may lead you into a trap. The trap of numbers. You may think that a calorie is a calorie, and this is the problem. Let's dive further into the subject. A calorie is nothing more than an energy measurement, and yes, all calories are equal in terms of the number that measures this energy that the body either uses or needs. They are equal as numbers. The question, though, is: are all calories the same? Numerically, they are, but in reality, they are not.

To understand this further, you need to examine the nutrients you receive from the food you consume and how you digest and metabolise them. These nutrients mainly belong to the following categories: protein, fat, and carbohydrates. For each of these elements, the body has a different way of breaking them down, digesting them, and absorbing the necessary nutrients it will use for energy. To metabolise them, the body uses energy, and this used energy differs for each category of nutrients.

For example, if the body needs to break down 100 calories of protein, it can only absorb 70, as it consumes 30 calories during digestion. This is called caloric availability. So, protein has a caloric availability of 70%. In comparison, fat has a caloric availability of 98%, and carbohydrates vary between 90% and 95%. The variation in this latter category is due to the complexity of the processing that carbohydrates have undergone during food preparation. If they are refined a lot, they can be broken down more easily.

Reviewing all of the above, you can understand that one calorie of protein is a product of a different way of digestion compared to those of fat or carbohydrates. In simpler terms, calories from a fizzy drink that contains sugar (carbohydrate) are absorbed more quickly and almost in their entirety than the calories from an egg, as the egg will need more time to be broken down into its nutrients and will consume more energy during this process.

This is why some people argue that protein consumption is better for weight loss. There are diets that promote this.

The question that arises now is, what about fat? Fat is necessary for the body, but it must not be consumed in excess. In addition, fat from animals may be more damaging to our health than fat from plants. To recognise the difference, you need to leave the fat at room temperature. Animal fat will remain solid, but fat from plants will be liquid. However, in every rule, there is an exception. Coconut oil is solid at room temperature.

Finally, as already mentioned, to maintain a healthy microbiome, you need to consume fibres. The minimum recommended consumption is 30 grams per day.

There are people who are consuming them in liquid form as a healthy drink because it is found that plants require more effort to be prepared, thus spending more time in your mouth. Chewing the food, however, is healthy as it stimulates the body and prepares it to receive the food, breaking it down into different elements and digesting the nutrients. This applies to all types of food, but plants require more effort. This is the reason that a number of nutritionists talk about the Mediterranean diet, as it consists of plants, olive oil, fruits, and lean meat.

Apply the Hippocratic rule: "*Let food be your medicine and medicine be your food.*"

To do so, you need to:

1. Eat a diverse range of food, as the different species require different nutrients to help their growth and be diverse themselves. In our modern diet, there is a lot of sugar used as preservatives. The overconsumption of it, can help the growth of one species that can dominate other species and this way you are out of balance. So, avoid sugar and any other sweeteners completely.

2. Eat a lot of vegetables and fruits with a high number of fibres to help the normal growth. The easier way to achieve this, is to make vegetable and fruit juices from raw vegetables and fruits. A number of people are able to do this because they have their own juicer machines. The specific family of bacteria benefits from such a diet and is known to be very beneficial in preventing intestinal inflammation. They thrive with this diet. In addition to the juices, your diet could include foods like beans, lentils, chickpeas, raspberries, apples, and bananas.

3. Eat fermented foods as they introduce healthy bacteria in our guts, like yoghurt (unsweetened) or sauerkraut (cabbage fermented).

4. Eat prebiotic and probiotic foods. Prebiotics are foods that promote good bacterial growth and probiotics are those that already contain beneficial bacteria.

Prebiotics are mainly food for the bacteria and not for us - such foods contain high fibre content, that pass the small intestine and the bacteria of the large intestine breaks them down. There are some indications that prebiotic foods can help the control of diabetes, heart disease and obesity.

5. Eat foods containing whole grains and ensure they are not refined. This way, you can reduce inflammation of your gut and improve gluten intolerance.
6. Have a plant-based diet and possible fruits rich in polyphenols. Polyphenols can be beneficial for the control of blood pressure, cholesterol levels, inflammation or even influence heart problems. Such foods are grapes, blueberries, broccoli, onions, almonds, cocoa and dark chocolate.
7. Apple cider vinegar can be beneficial to blood sugar control and weight balance, as it is thought that it reduces the insulin resistance.
8. There are reports that curcumin (element found in turmeric), red wine and coffee, can stimulate autophagy. *Do not forget that these are results of experiments made in laboratories and not seen on humans.*

> **PLEASE CONTACT YOUR PHYSICIAN FOR FURTHER INFORMATION.**

Include regular exercise in any diet; this is very important. It is necessary to prevent unwanted changes in the body during dieting. When weight loss begins, especially when autophagy occurs, the body can lose muscle tissue. To avoid this, you need to continue exercising to aid in muscle recovery and growth.

Taking all of this into consideration, the need for persistence and necessary action can change our beliefs about food.

The minimum amount of time needed to rewire the brain is estimated to be three months. This is the duration during which you must maintain extreme discipline if you want to establish a new habit. You must change your diet.

The word "diet" reminds me of a story from my time in medical school. It was during my surgical rotation training when I was asked to go and admit a patient. This individual was scheduled to undergo a cholecystectomy (removal of the gallbladder), and it was necessary to reduce their BMI (Body Mass Index) because the instruments available were not long enough to retract and visualise the organ that needed to be removed. A strict low-calorie diet had been prescribed during a previous consultation. After reviewing the patient's file, I went to see them. I conducted a thorough examination, including recalculating their BMI. To my surprise, I found that it was higher than before. I asked if they had followed the prescribed diet, and the response I received was:

"Yes, doctor, I ate everything that was written on the paper given to me."

I had my doubts, so I inquired about the daily food that had been consumed. The response I received was another surprise:

"In the morning, I ate my usual breakfast and then consumed the diet that was written on the paper given to me. At lunchtime, I had my usual lunch and added the prescribed diet. At dinnertime, I prepared my regular dinner and followed the instructed diet."

When I asked the patient what they believed the purpose of the diet was, I received the following answer:

"Usually, I take my medication after eating, and since the diet was given to me by the hospital, I considered it to be like medication, so I took it after meals. Why are you asking all of this? Have I made a mistake?"

Mentally, I was astonished, and I realised that there was a communication issue. I explained how a diet works and how it should be followed. The operation was postponed once again until the desired BMI was achieved.

Therefore, a diet is not a medication; it is a way of life. It is necessary to educate yourself about different foods and how to eat healthily at all times. This helps restore balance to the body.

Hippocrates once said:

"What preserves health is an isomeric distribution and exact mixing of the forces (isonomy) of dry, wet, cold, sweet, bitter, sour and salty. A disease is caused by the dominance of one (monarchy). The cure is achieved by restoring the disturbed balance, by the method of the opposite of the excess force."

To achieve an improvement in our body chemistry, as well as our physical and mental health, we need to go through these 5 M's and work hard.

Nutrition problems are influenced by your physical needs, but they are also connected to your mind. Part of this connection is related to your microbiome, as these bacteria influence your body's chemistry. The other reason is the habits you create. To achieve the goal of a permanent solution to your high BMI, you need to find the reason why you want to fulfil this goal. In other words, you have to find the WHY. If you can honestly and openly answer the question, "Why do I want to lose weight?", you will be able to find the path that leads you to your lighthouse.

RECIPES

Below you can find some low-calorie recipes for potential diets. These recipes are for one or two people and have approximately 500 calories per serving, as well as a low glycaemic index.

Grilled Chicken and Quinoa Salad

(serves 2, approximately 500 calories per serving)

Ingredients

- 2 boneless, skinless chicken breasts
- ½ cup uncooked quinoa
- ½ cup chopped cucumber
- ½ cup chopped cherry tomatoes
- ¼ red onion, thinly sliced
- ¼ cup chopped fresh parsley
- ¼ cup chopped fresh mint
- 2 tablespoons extra-virgin olive oil
- 2 tablespoons fresh lemon juice
- Salt and pepper to taste

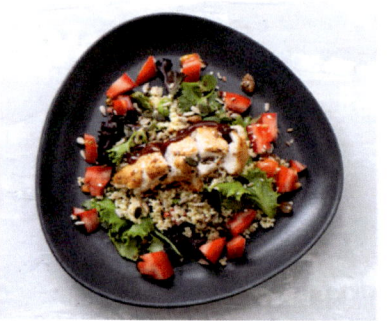

Instructions

1. Cook the quinoa according to package instructions. Once cooked, fluff with a fork and set aside to cool.
2. Pre-heat the grill to medium-high heat. Season the chicken breasts with salt and pepper. Grill the chicken for 5-6 minutes per side, or until cooked through. Remove from heat and let it rest for 5 minutes before slicing.

3. In a large bowl, combine the cooked quinoa, cucumber, cherry tomatoes, red onion, parsley, and mint.
4. In a small bowl, whisk together the olive oil, lemon juice, salt, and pepper.
5. Add the sliced chicken to the quinoa salad and drizzle the dressing over the top. Toss to combine.

This recipe provides a good balance of protein and carbohydrates, with the quinoa serving as a high-protein, low-glycaemic index grain. The vegetables also contribute fibre and nutrients to the dish. Just make sure to adjust the portion sizes to fit your individual calorie needs.

Baked Salmon and Sweet Potato

(serves 1, approximately 500 calories per serving)

Ingredients

- 1 salmon fillet (4-6 ounces)
- 1 medium sweet potato
- ½ tablespoon olive oil
- Salt and pepper to taste
- ½ teaspoon garlic powder
- ½ teaspoon paprika
- ½ teaspoon dried thyme

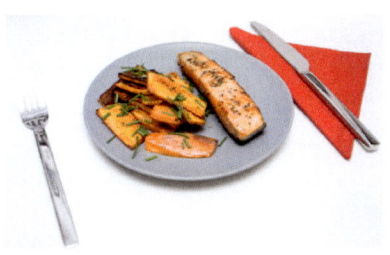

Instructions

1. Preheat the oven to 400°F (200°C).
2. Wash the sweet potato and pierce it all over with a fork. Place it on a baking sheet and bake for 45-50 minutes, or until tender.
3. While the sweet potato is baking, brush the salmon fillet with olive oil and season with salt, pepper, garlic powder, paprika, and dried thyme.

4. Once the sweet potato is done, remove it from the oven and reduce the temperature to 375°F (190°C). Push the sweet potato to one side of the baking sheet and place the salmon fillet on the other side. Bake for 12-15 minutes, or until the salmon is cooked to your desired level of doneness.
5. Serve the salmon and sweet potato hot, garnished with fresh herbs or a squeeze of lemon juice if desired.

This recipe provides a great source of protein and healthy fats from the salmon, as well as complex carbohydrates and fibre from the sweet potato. Both foods have a low glycaemic index, which means they would not cause a rapid spike in blood sugar levels. If you need additional calories, you could add a side salad or steamed vegetables to the meal.

Grilled Tofu and Vegetable Kabobs
(serves 1, approximately 500 calories per serving)

Ingredients

- ½ block of firm tofu, pressed and cut into cubes
- 1 small zucchini, sliced into rounds
- 1 small yellow squash, sliced into rounds
- 1 small red onion, cut into wedges
- 1 small red bell pepper, cut into chunks
- 1 small green bell pepper, cut into chunks
- 2 tablespoons olive oil
- 1 tablespoon balsamic vinegar
- 1 teaspoon Dijon mustard

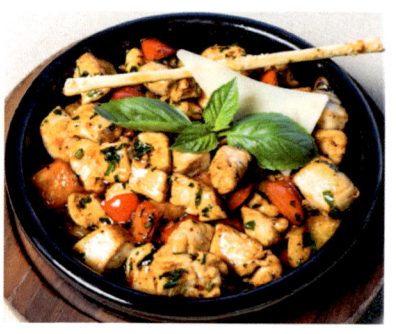

- ½ teaspoon dried oregano
- Salt and pepper to taste

Instructions

1. Pre-heat the grill to medium-high heat.
2. Thread the tofu and vegetables onto skewers in a desired pattern.
3. In a small bowl, whisk together the olive oil, balsamic vinegar, Dijon mustard, dried oregano, salt, and pepper.
4. Brush the kabobs with the marinade, reserving any extra for later.
5. Grill the kabobs for 8-10 minutes, or until the vegetables are tender and the tofu is lightly browned, turning once.
6. Serve the kabobs hot, drizzled with any remaining marinade.

This recipe provides a great source of plant-based protein from the tofu, as well as fibre and nutrients from the vegetables. The marinade adds flavour without adding extra sugar, and the low glycaemic index of the vegetables and tofu helps to keep blood sugar levels stable. You could serve this dish with a side salad or a small portion of brown rice or quinoa if you need additional calories.

Turkey and Sweet Potato Chili

(serves 1, approximately 500 calories per serving)

Ingredients

- 4 ounces ground turkey
- 1 small, sweet potato, peeled and diced
- ½ small onion, diced
- ½ red bell pepper, diced
- 1 garlic clove, minced
- ½ tablespoon olive oil

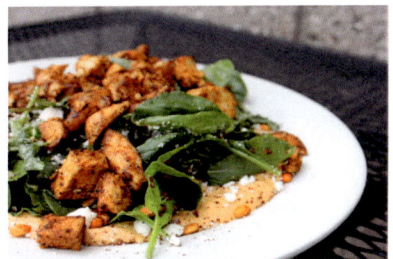

- ½ tablespoon chili powder
- ½ teaspoon ground cumin
- ¼ teaspoon smoked paprika
- ¼ teaspoon dried oregano
- ¼ teaspoon salt
- ¼ teaspoon black pepper
- ½ cup canned diced tomatoes
- ½ cup low-sodium chicken broth
- *Optional toppings: shredded cheddar cheese, sliced green onions*

Instructions

1. Heat the olive oil in a medium saucepan over medium-high heat.
2. Add the ground turkey and cook, breaking it up with a spatula, until browned and cooked through, about 5-7 minutes.
3. Add the sweet potato, onion, bell pepper, and garlic to the pan. Cook, stirring occasionally, until the vegetables are tender, about 5-7 minutes.
4. Add the chili powder, cumin, smoked paprika, oregano, salt, and black pepper to the pan. Stir to combine and cook for 1-2 minutes, until fragrant.
5. Add the canned diced tomatoes and chicken broth to the pan. Bring the mixture to a simmer and cook for 15-20 minutes, or until the sweet potatoes are tender and the flavours have melded together.
6. Serve the chili hot, garnished with shredded cheddar cheese and sliced green onions if desired.

This recipe provides a great source of protein from the ground turkey, as well as complex carbohydrates and fibre from the sweet potato. The low glycaemic index of the sweet potato helps to keep blood sugar levels stable, while the spices add flavour without adding extra sugar. You could pair this dish with a side salad or a small portion of brown rice or quinoa if you need additional calories.

Grilled Steak and Asparagus Salad

(serves 1, approximately 500 calories per serving)

Ingredients

- 4 ounces flank steak
- ½ tablespoon olive oil
- Salt and pepper to taste
- ½ pound asparagus, trimmed
- ½ small red onion, thinly sliced
- ¼ cup cherry tomatoes, halved
- ¼ cup crumbled feta cheese
- ½ tablespoon balsamic vinegar
- ½ tablespoon honey
- 1 teaspoon Dijon mustard
- ½ teaspoon dried thyme

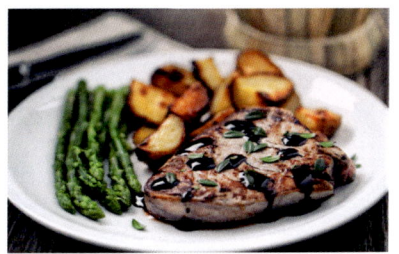

Instructions

1. Preheat the grill to medium-high heat.
2. Brush the flank steak with olive oil and season with salt and pepper. Grill the steak for 3-4 minutes per side, or until cooked to your desired level of doneness. Remove from the heat and let it rest for 5 minutes before slicing.
3. While the steak is resting, grill the asparagus for 3-4 minutes, or until tender and lightly charred.
4. In a small bowl, whisk together the balsamic vinegar, honey, Dijon mustard, dried thyme, salt, and pepper.

5. In a large bowl, combine the sliced steak, grilled asparagus, red onion, cherry tomatoes, and crumbled feta cheese.
6. Drizzle the dressing over the salad and toss to combine.

This recipe provides a good balance of protein and carbohydrates, with the steak serving as a high-protein source and the asparagus providing complex carbohydrates and fibre. The low glycaemic index of the asparagus helps to keep blood sugar levels stable. The dressing adds flavour without adding extra sugar, and the feta cheese provides a source of calcium.

You could serve this dish with a small side of whole grain bread or quinoa if you need additional calories.

Chicken Breast with Quinoa
(Meal serves 1 person and contains around 500 calories per serving)

Ingredients

- 4 oz boneless, skinless chicken breast
- ½ cup quinoa
- 1 cup water
- ½ cup green beans, trimmed
- ½ red bell pepper, sliced
- ½ tbsp coconut oil
- ½ tbsp soy sauce
- ½ tbsp honey
- ½ clove garlic, minced
- Salt and pepper to taste

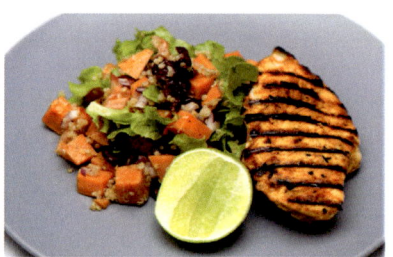

Instructions

1. Rinse the quinoa in a fine-mesh strainer and place it in a medium saucepan with 1 cup of water. Bring to a boil, and then reduce heat to low and cover. Simmer for about 15 minutes or until the water is absorbed and the quinoa is tender.
2. Preheat a grill pan or outdoor grill to medium-high heat.
3. Season the chicken breast with salt and pepper.
4. Grill the chicken breast for 6-8 minutes per side, or until cooked through.
5. While the chicken is grilling, steam the green beans in a steamer basket for about 5-7 minutes, or until they are tender but still crisp.
6. In a small saucepan, melt the coconut oil over low heat. Add the soy sauce, honey, and garlic and stir to combine. Remove from heat.
7. In a large bowl, combine the cooked quinoa, green beans, and sliced red bell pepper.
8. Once the chicken is cooked, slice it into strips and add it to the bowl with the quinoa and vegetables.
9. Drizzle the sauce over the top of the mixture and toss to combine.
10. Serve immediately.

This recipe provides a good balance of protein, complex carbohydrates, and healthy fats, making it a great choice for bodybuilders. The chicken breast is a lean source of protein, while the quinoa and green beans provide complex carbohydrates and fibre. The low glycaemic index of this recipe comes from the use of quinoa instead of high-glycaemic grains like white rice or pasta. The sauce is made with coconut oil, which is a healthy source of medium-chain triglycerides (MCTs) that can help boost energy levels during workouts.

VEGETARIAN RECIPES

Vegetarian Quinoa Salad
(serves 1 person and contains around 500 calories per serving)

Ingredients

- ½ cup quinoa
- 1 cup water
- ½ red bell pepper, diced
- ½ yellow bell pepper, diced
- ½ cucumber, diced
- ¼ red onion, diced
- 1 tablespoon chopped fresh parsley
- 1 tablespoon chopped fresh mint
- 1 tablespoon extra-virgin olive oil
- 1 tablespoon red wine vinegar
- Salt and pepper to taste

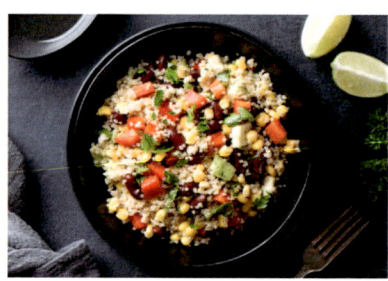

Instructions

1. Rinse the quinoa in a fine-mesh strainer and place it in a medium saucepan with 1 cup of water. Bring to a boil, then reduce heat to low and cover. Simmer for about 15 minutes or until the water is absorbed and the quinoa is tender.
2. Fluff the quinoa with a fork and let it cool to room temperature.
3. In a large bowl, combine the cooked quinoa, diced bell peppers, cucumber, red onion, parsley, and mint.
4. In a small bowl, whisk together the olive oil, red wine vinegar, salt, and pepper.
5. Pour the dressing over the quinoa salad and toss to combine.
6. Serve immediately or cover and refrigerate until ready to serve.

This recipe is packed with nutrients and contains a good balance of protein, fibre, and healthy fats. Quinoa is a great source of protein and fibre, while the vegetables provide vitamins and minerals. The low glycaemic index of this recipe comes from the use of quinoa instead of high-glycaemic grains like white rice or pasta.

Vegetarian Quinoa Salad with Sweet Potato

(serves 1 person and contains around 500 calories per serving)

Ingredients

- ½ cup quinoa
- 1 cup water
- ½ medium sweet potato, peeled and diced
- ½ cup broccoli florets
- ¼ red onion, diced
- ½ tablespoon olive oil
- ½ tablespoon balsamic vinegar
- Salt and pepper to taste
- ¼ cup crumbled feta cheese (optional)

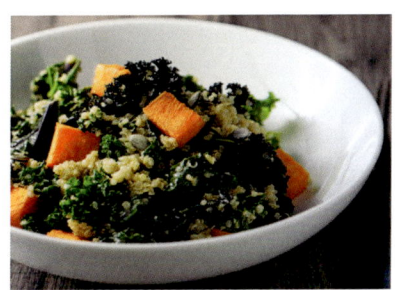

Instructions:

1. Rinse the quinoa in a fine-mesh strainer and place it in a medium saucepan with 1 cup of water. Bring to a boil, and then reduce heat to low and cover. Simmer for about 15 minutes or until the water is absorbed and the quinoa is tender.
2. Preheat the oven to 400°F (200°C).
3. Toss the diced sweet potato and broccoli florets with the olive oil and season with salt and pepper.
4. Spread the sweet potato and broccoli on a baking sheet and roast for 15-20 minutes, or until tender.

5. In a large bowl, combine the cooked quinoa, roasted sweet potato and broccoli, and diced red onion.
6. In a small bowl, whisk together the balsamic vinegar, salt, and pepper.
7. Pour the dressing over the quinoa salad and toss to combine.
8. Sprinkle feta cheese over the top, if desired.
9. Serve immediately or cover and refrigerate until ready to serve.

This recipe is a great source of complex carbohydrates, fibre, and vitamins. The quinoa provides a complete source of protein, while the sweet potato and broccoli are rich in vitamins A and C. The low glycaemic index of this recipe comes from the use of quinoa and sweet potato, which are both low-glycaemic carbohydrates. The addition of feta cheese provides some healthy fats and protein, but you can omit it if you prefer a vegan option.

The question is, what is needed for you to manage and control your BMI?

Is it knowledge?

Is it training?

Is it specialisation in cooking?

Discipline, **Persistence** and **Focus** are the answers.

If you ask me if this is easy, I can tell you that it needs a lot of work, discipline, concentration, persistence, and belief in yourself, but it is possible.

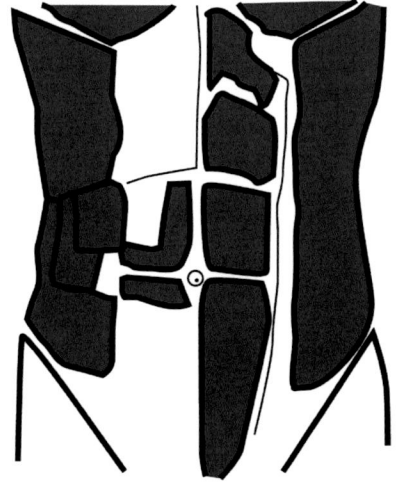

> **PLEASE DO NOT FORGET THAT THIS IS ONLY FOR EDUCATIONAL PURPOSES AND IF THERE ARE ANY HEALTH ISSUES, YOU SHOULD ASK YOUR OWN DOCTOR FOR FURTHER ADVICE AND TREATMENT. THIS IS NOT A MEDICAL CONSULTATION.**

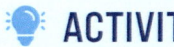 **ACTIVITY**

From all the previous activities you have undertaken, you must already know a lot about your current state, the treatment methods you have followed, and your goals. Now, you need to put all of this together and delve deep within yourself to answer the following questions:

1. Where are you?
2. Where do you want to go?
3. Why do you need to do this?
4. What do you have to do to achieve change?
5. How will you do it?
6. Once you are calm and settled, choose one goal to pursue and stick with it.

Analyse your habits and focus on the necessary actions for a positive outcome while eliminating any negative thoughts. Get rid of any distractions.

IMPLEMENTATION

In this section, we will go into more detail and describe the potential solution. We will delve deeper and explore how the 5 M's can be implemented. This is the time when the fruits of my journey can assist you. Allow me to use my experience as a bridge to bring you the solution, which I call the resurrection. I will describe how I found ways to manage all the difficulties I faced.

Anyone who has an "unknown" problem initially panics and sinks into the dark abyss. I have experienced this myself, but I fought back and climbed back into the light. I know that many of you are going through similar dark experiences, so please allow me to offer myself and my services to help you overcome this negativity. Together, we can emerge from the abyss and return to the light.

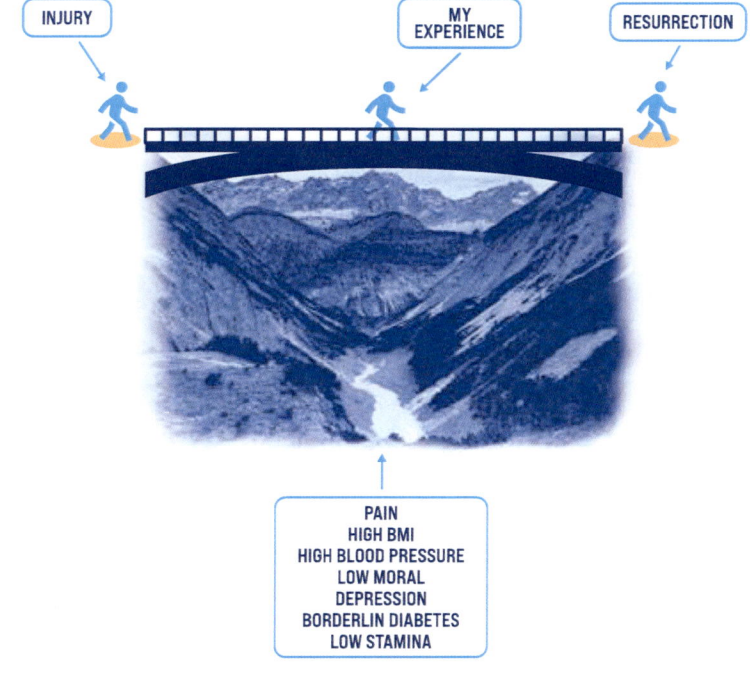

I am here to share with you my experiences and serve you based on the following factors. Firstly, I am one of you, as I have lived through the experiences of being a chronic back pain sufferer for the last 25 years. Secondly, I have professional experience, with 39 years as an Orthopaedic Surgeon. Utilising these, along with a great deal of research and experimentation, I managed to improve my symptoms.

When someone is suffering from chronic low back pain, their goal is to control it and live a normal life, preferably without symptoms. Unfortunately, the latter is not possible, so the realistic goal is for you to live a life with long periods of normality without symptoms.

This is why I am sharing my journey with you, as this is what I have managed to achieve. I live a life with long periods without symptoms, although I am aware that the "dragon" is still there, dormant, and can awaken with any misstep.

I am here to share my experiences, strategies, the steps I took, and the proposed solutions that any of you can do to improve your health. We will follow the 5 M's strategy.

> **ONCE MORE I AM STRESSING THAT, FIRSTLY, ALL INFORMATION GIVEN IS BASED ON MY OWN EXPERIENCES AND IT SERVES AN EDUCATIONAL PURPOSE. FROM THIS, YOU ARE ADVISED TO KEEP THE SECTIONS THAT RESONATE WITH YOU. NOTICE THAT THIS IS NOT A MEDICAL CONSULTATION OR ADVICE.**

MOTION

I already mentioned that I became overweight. Following my back injury and as I went through the initial immobilisation, to the degree I was allowed by the hospital's needs, and as physiotherapy was not available to me due to my very busy schedule (I never had time; This latter is the silliest statement someone has as an excuse. I urge you to forget this phrase. YOU HAVE AND YOU MUST HAVE TIME FOR YOURSELF), but also, I was not referred by my own doctor. I reached a weight of 127kg when my upper limit for a normal BMI for my somatotype should be 85kg. I was classified as obese. My mouth seems to have been doing overtime mainly next to the fridge. To avoid long-term medicinal treatment, I became captain of my ship.

I started walking. I bought a pair of trainers with shock-absorbing soles and insoles. Don't forget that discs are shock absorbers, and they need help. This external shock absorption also helped my other joints. Initially, my walks were short and gradually the distance increased. When I reached 8 miles, I started to time myself and see if I could do the distance faster. During this period, I developed knee pain as a result of the stupid accelerations in the early stages, while I was carrying a lot of weight. Please do not repeat this mistake.

When I found that I was getting comfortable with this level of motion and because my enthusiasm started to evaporate, I tried to find ways to persevere and sustain my activity. I subscribed to a local gym and managed to strike a deal to include a session with a trainer for one hour each week. That helped my motivation and my confidence a lot.

My knowledge of anatomy helped me discuss with the trainer the possible beneficial exercises to achieve my goal of improving my muscles and supporting my back. My gym sessions initially were limited to 30-45 minutes once a week, and when I reached an hour, I asked for the trainer's support. The frequency increased slowly and finally, I reached a daily presence in the gym, although this was only for half an hour every morning before work, incorporating swimming in my attempt to utilise water and offload my spine.

I lost weight, my blood pressure went down to normal limits, and my back pain episodes are very, very rare. Despite this, my BMI still was not fully improving. So, I had to do something more, and we will see about it later on.

As you can see in a couple of paragraphs, I included my whole mobility plan. Was it though so easy? No, certainly it was not. It took me two years to achieve my goal, and this was because I was not fully aware that I had to add more elements to fight the back pain. I was not aware of the rest of the M's.

But let us concentrate on motion again.

Why do you need to stay mobile? Movement helps your thinking, your confidence, as well as the hormonal system of your body.

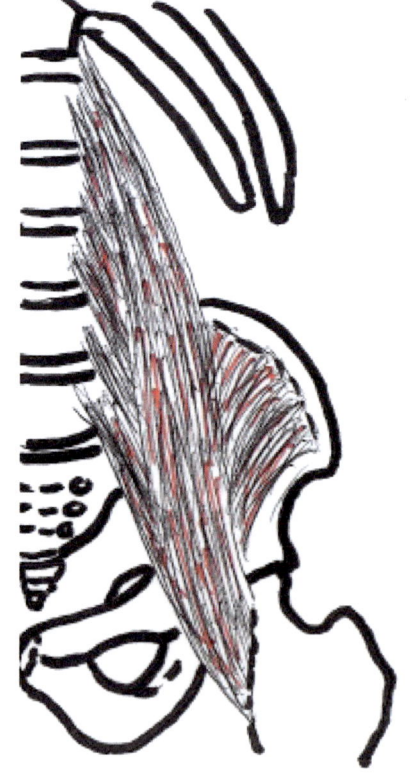

What is the goal? Mechanically, you need to become more flexible and be able to use the muscles as additional shock absorbers, as well as stabilisers of your spine. To stabilise your spine, you need to have strong core muscles. Flexibility, on the other hand, has to be extended not only to the spine but also to the hip joints, as the upper part of the thigh bone (femur) is attached to the spine with muscles, and the most important of them is the iliopsoas, as seen in the drawing.

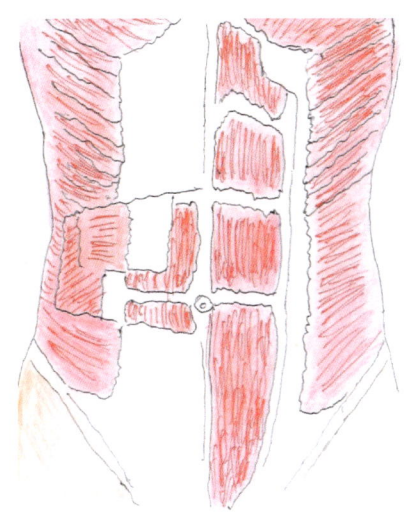

When people hear about core muscle strengthening exercises, they often focus solely on the abdominal muscles, specifically the six-pack muscles known as the rectus abdominis. However, it is important to remember that there are other muscles involved, such as the lateral abdominal muscles, which have fibres that run either obliquely or horizontally. Crunches, which target the front abdominals (the six-pack), are not effective on their own since they only work the muscles with fibres running from top to bottom. It is crucial to strengthen all the muscles in the core, so a combination of exercises needs to be incorporated.

So, what kind of exercises do you need to do? How often do we need to do them? Which muscles are involved in every exercise? What is the overall benefit? What time of the day do we need to do them?

There is a certain way for you to prepare for your exercises. Firstly, you need to learn to concentrate on your breathing, then you need to warm up, and the sequence of stretching and working out has to be followed.

Why breathing, you may ask.

For the following reasons:

1. You need oxygen to arrive at your muscles during your workout.
2. Your mind and body work together, so relaxation is fully understood by your brain, and this helps the release of muscle

tension when necessary (breathe in = tension of muscles, breathe out = relaxation).

3. When the body has less air in the lungs, it is getting more flexible, although the muscles are not well oxygenated.
4. You are getting into a rhythm, as breathing can become "music in your ears."

To perform any exercises and increase the muscle response, you need to warm up. A warm muscle is more flexible. You are fighting stiffness, so you need flexible muscles. This technique helps the blood flow through the muscle. Warming up could happen with extra simple light exercises or simple movements. In some cases, a warm bath could be considered.

Stretching gives flexibility to the muscle, so that is essential before you do any strengthening exercises. A stretched flexible muscle is able to move a greater distance than a short, stiff muscle. In addition, a short, stiff muscle is prone to injuries as the range of activity is limited. An injury caused by the overstretching of a stiff, short muscle can result in prolonged symptoms, as in some cases, back pain becomes worse. When you exercise and stretch your muscle, it would be beneficial to maintain this stretched position for five to ten breaths.

Talking now about frequency, initially it is evident to all that you have to start light, and you could divide some of the exercises in the morning and some others before bed. This way, you may find that you are going to achieve good results. In both cases, a warm bath or shower will help you have good muscle recovery and, on top of that, a nice sleep after the evening session. Please do not overdo it.

When your mobility improves and you start the strengthening exercises, it will be better if you perform them once every three days. That will give enough time for your muscles to recover.

So now let's concentrate on some of the exercises. Wear comfortable clothing.

Below you will see some of the exercises you can do at home (you will need a well-padded yoga mat – I found that the slim one was too thin for me, and my knees were hurting.

TERMINOLOGY

Isometric: a muscle contraction without the result of movement.

Isotonic: a muscle contraction producing movement.

Dorsal area: the back of the body.

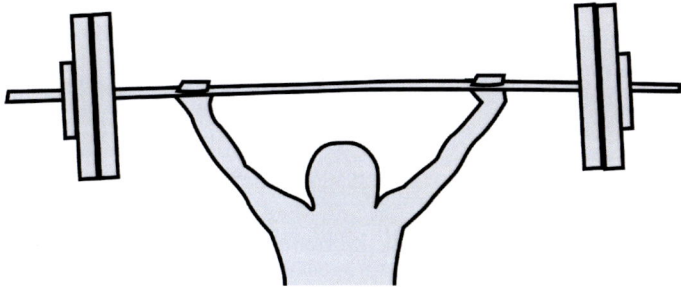

EXERCISES

The following exercises are in general simple. You can perform them in your own home, using your own furniture and even wearing your everyday clothes, as you will see. You don't have to own any specific equipment or to be member of any specific expensive club. As you can see, I am able to perform all of them without any expense at all.

In case you want to wear comfortable clothes, have a yoga mat or even go to gym, I will not fault you. It will be much more comfortable, I understand. Please do what is best for you.

Photos illustrate the sequence of positions you have to take.

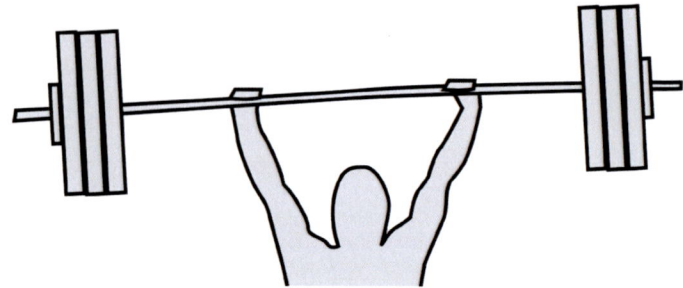

A. HAMSTRING STRETCHING

The purpose of the exercise is to stretch the muscles at the back of the legs. This exercise can be done by lying on the floor or by using different stools or supports. Below, you can see the exercise being performed by lying on the floor.

You may perform this exercise with the knee of the opposite leg either bent or straight, as seen in the pictures.

1. Lie on the floor.
2. Bend the knees and then extend one of the legs and lift it in the air.
3. Support it preferably from the area of the calf, as this way you stretch the back of the knee (not demonstrated in these pictures).
4. Keep this position for about 30-60 seconds (shorter time in the beginning) and control your breathing.
5. Repeat 5-10 times (less in the initial stages).
6. Repeat the same with the other leg.

WITH KNEE BENT

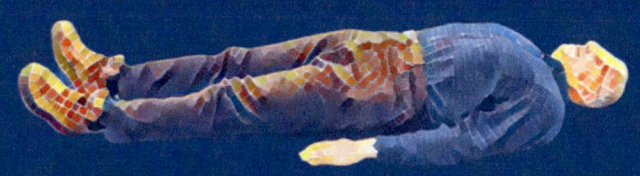

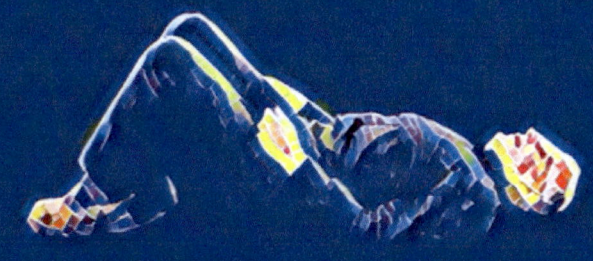

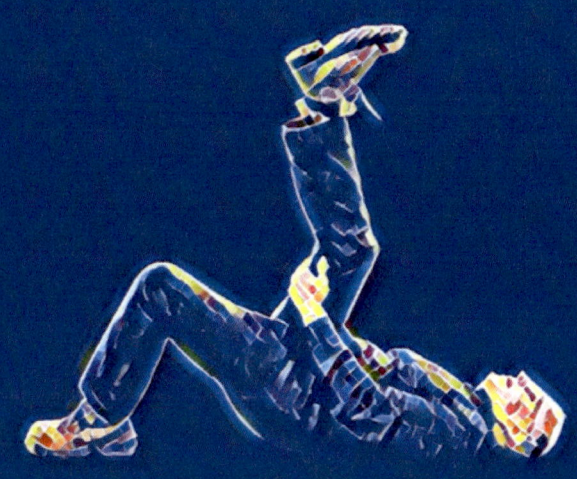

WITH KNEE STRAIGHT

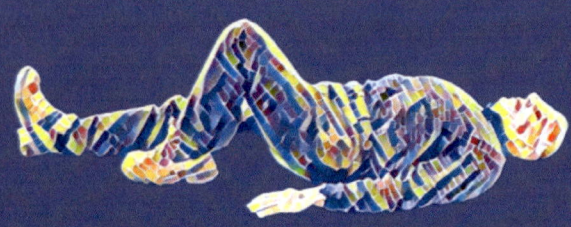

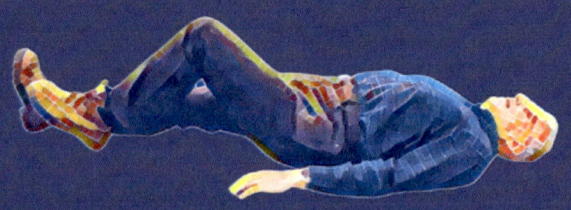

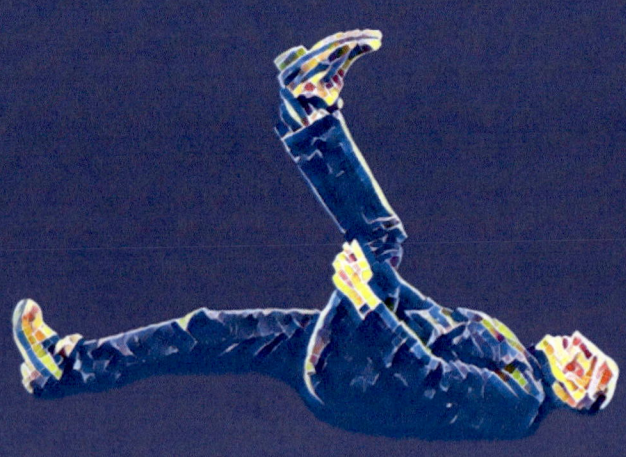

If you use a stool or chair, it could be easier.

1. Place the heel of one of the legs on a stool or chair, about half a meter high.
2. Keep the knee straight.
3. Bend the body at the hip joint by leaning forward.
4. Feel the stretch at the back of the leg.
5. Hold this position for about 30-60 seconds (shorter time in the beginning) and control your breathing.
6. Repeat for 5-10 times (less in the initial stages).
7. Repeat the same with the other leg.

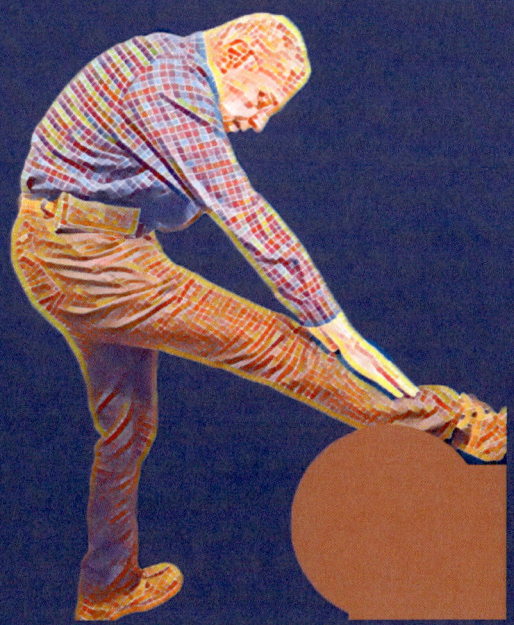

B. PELVIC TILT

1. Lie on your back (on the yoga mattress).
2. Bend your knees and keep your feet on the floor.
3. Tighten your abdominal muscles.
4. Press your back against the floor.
5. Hold this position for 6-10 seconds, gradually increasing to 10-30 seconds, then relax.
6. Complete three sets of 10-15 repetitions.

The aim is to make isotonic contractions of the abdominal muscles, while stretching the dorsal muscles of the spine, at the same time. This exercise also stretches the iliopsoas muscle.

LYING

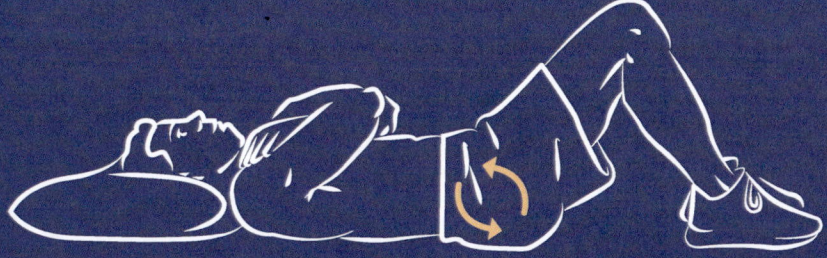

STANDING

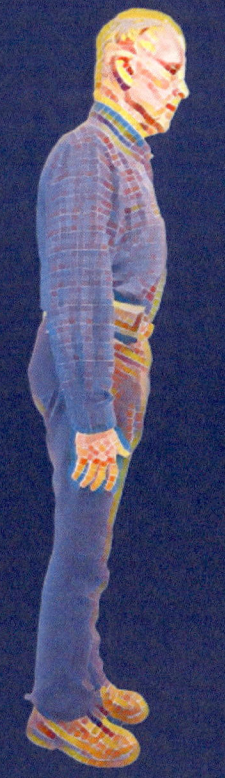
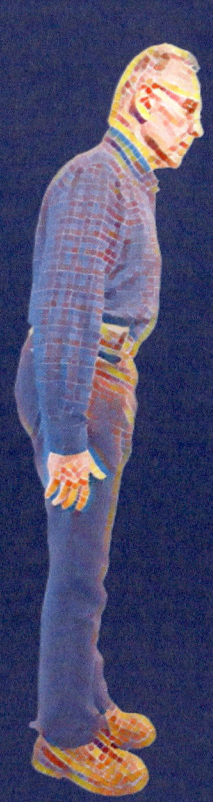

C. PARTIAL CURL

1. Stay on the floor lying on your back with knees bent and feet on the floor as above.
2. Tighten your abdominal muscles.
3. Bend your neck so your chin moves towards your chest.
4. Stretch your arms out in front of you.
5. Curl your upper body so your shoulders do not touch the floor.
6. Maintain this position for 5-10 seconds and relax.
7. Do 3 sets of 10-15 repetitions.

This is a strengthening exercise. The main active muscle is rectus abdominis (six-pack muscle). Lateral abdominal muscles are activated too, to a smaller degree.

With exercises like this one, you stabilise your spine on the pelvis.

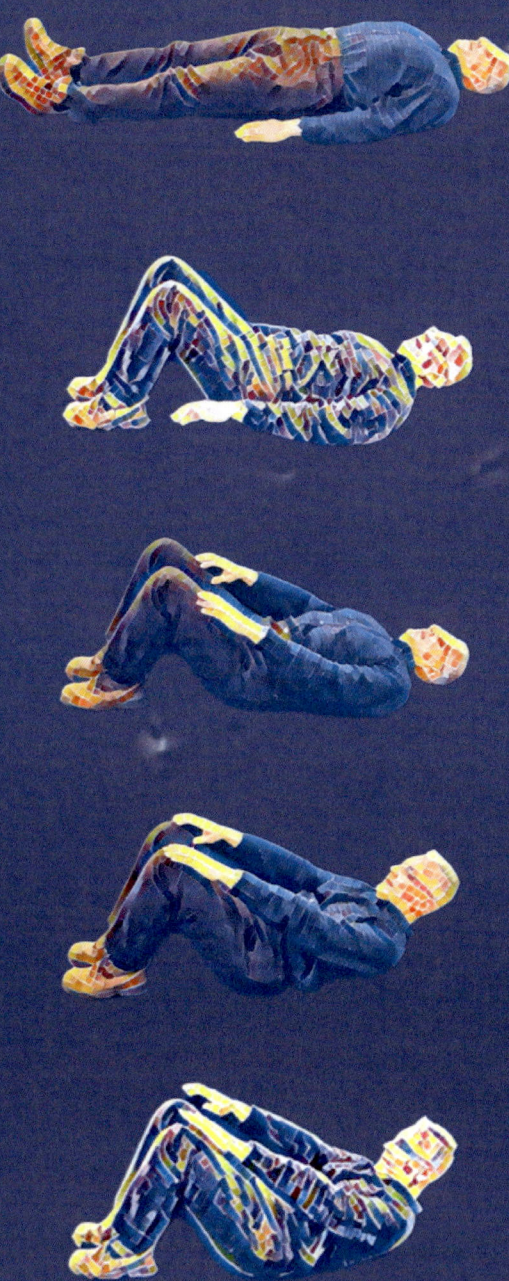

D. GLUTEAL STRETCH

1. Stay on the floor, lying on your back.
2. Keep one leg straight on the floor.
3. Bend the other knee towards your chest.
4. You will feel your gluteal (buttock) muscles stretching, as well as the muscles at the bottom of the spine and the back of the straight leg.
5. Hold this position for 20-60 seconds or for 5-10 breaths.
6. Repeat on the opposite side.
7. Do three sets of 10-15 repetitions.

The movements during this exercise need to be gradual. During the initial stages, you may find that the range of movement at the hip joint is not full. Do not worry. Slowly, this will improve.

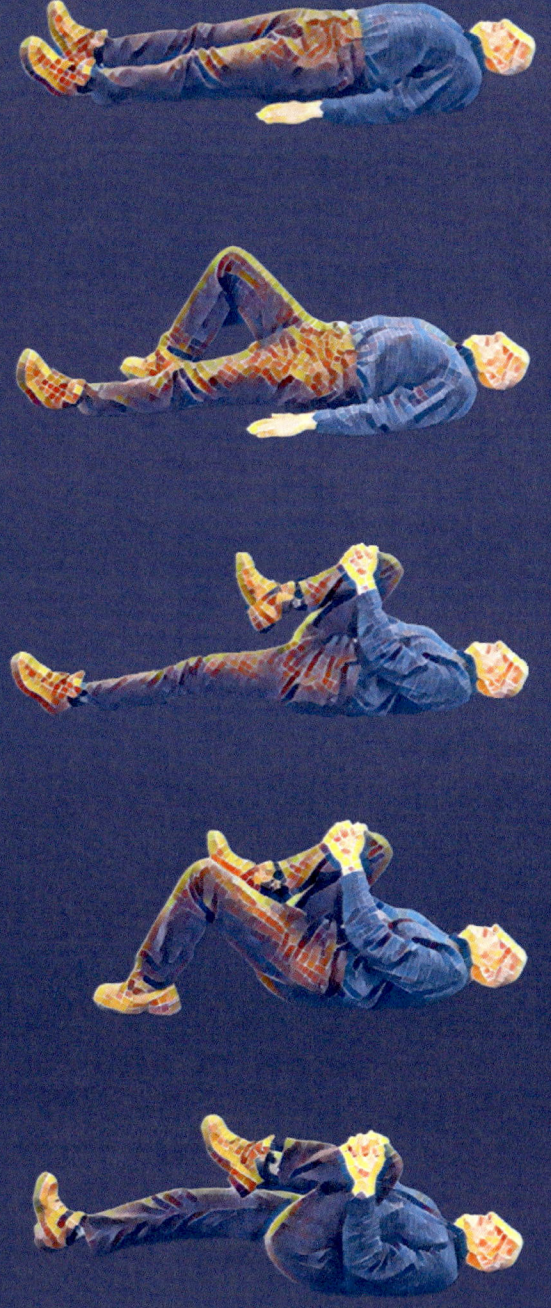

E. MODIFIED/ALTERNATIVE GLUTEAL STRETCH

(Keep position for 10-30 seconds. Repeat 3-5 times per leg 10-20 times)

MODIFIED

1. Keep the position as described in the previous section.
2. Flex the knee as before but add cross-leg rotation.
3. As you hold this knee with your opposite hand, keep rotating and pushing it toward the floor on the opposite side.
4. Feel the stretching of the gluteal (buttock) and hip piriformis (lateral aspect rotator) muscles.

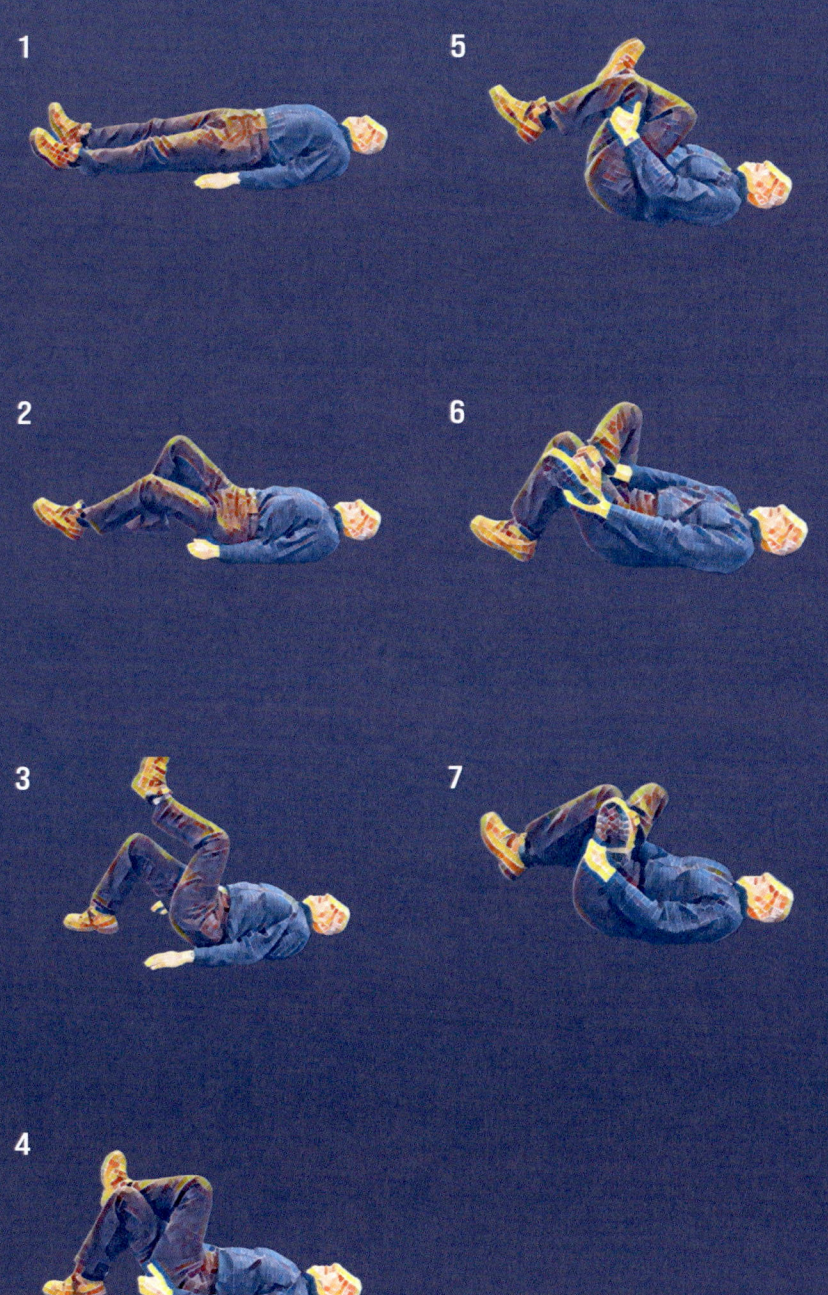

ALTERNATIVE

1. The same exercise can be done with the person facing down, kneeling on the floor. One leg should be straight on the floor, and the other leg should be crossed straight under the body on the opposite side, with the knee flexed.
2. The arms need to be extended straight forward as the person presses themselves down.
3. Stretching of the gluteal (buttock), piriformis (lateral hip muscles) at the flexed and rotated leg, and quadriceps (front thigh muscle), iliopsoas (muscle linking hip, pelvis, and spine), quadratus (dorsal muscle stabilising spine on pelvis), and lateral abdominal muscles are stretched on the extended leg.
4. Repeat the exercise with the other leg.
5. Take 5-10 breaths.

IMPLEMENTATION 135

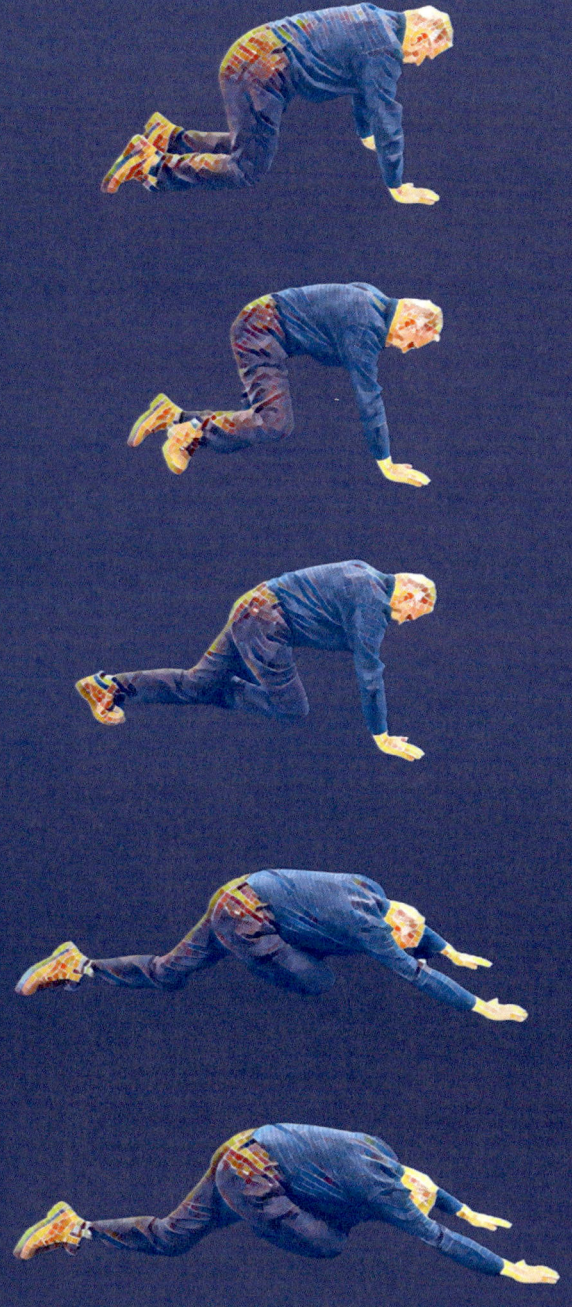

F. STRETCHING OF LOWER BACK

1. Lie on your back.
2. Bend both legs at the hip joints.
3. Put your hands behind the knees.
4. Bend the knees.
5. Pull the thighs towards your chest and let the knees almost touch your face.
6. Feel the stretching of the lower back muscles.
7. Maintain the position for 5-10 breaths.
8. Repeat 10-20 times.

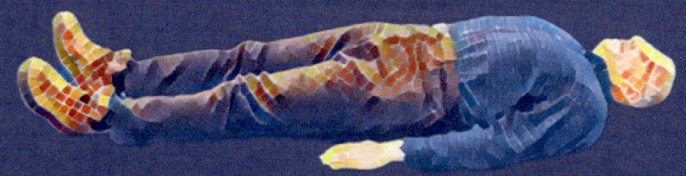

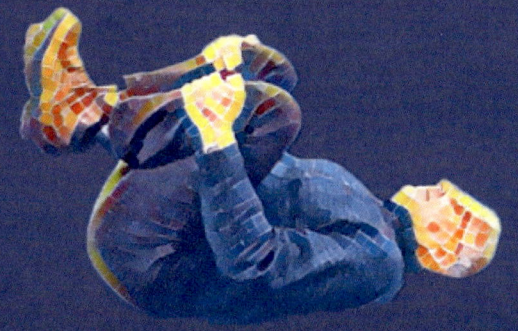

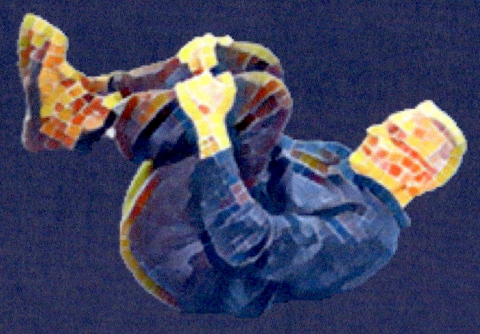

G. STRETCHING OF LOWER BACK AND LATERAL ABDOMINAL MUSCLES

1. Lying down on your back.
2. Flex hips and knees but keep feet on the floor.
3. Extend the arms to the sides.
4. Rotate the knees together to one side, trying to touch the floor with the side of the knee at the direction you are rotating. If knees rotate towards right, the lateral side of the right knee has to touch the floor, or one crossing over the other, as you rotate the pelvis. During the exercise concentrate on breathing as you need the rhythm. In addition, during exhaling you can achieve more rotational movement. You can either keep the opposite arm to the rotation extended to stabilise yourself and achieve a greater muscle stretch, while the other could be under your head.
5. Feel the stretching of the lateral muscles in the lower back, as well as the lateral hip muscles.
6. Hold the position for 5-10 breaths.
7. Complete 3-5 sets, with 10-20 repetitions.
8. Repeat the same steps for the opposite side.

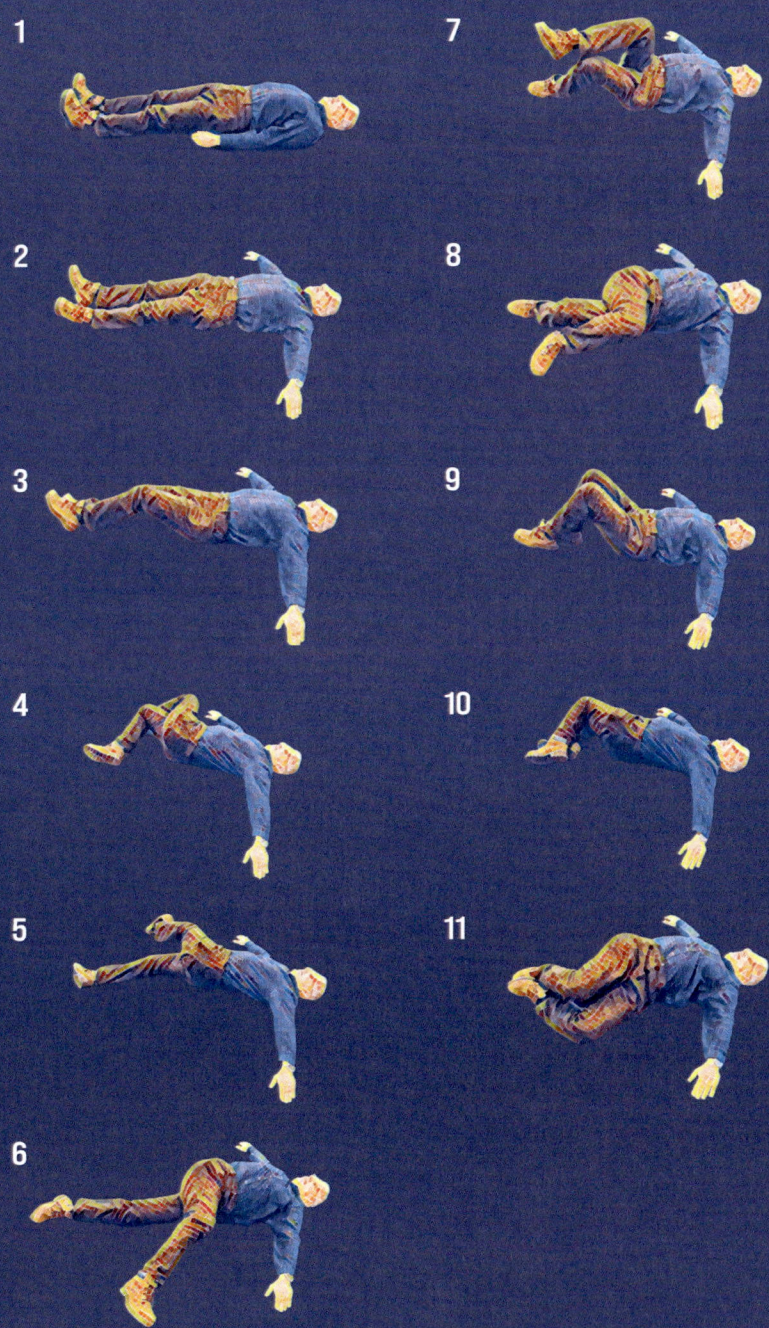

H. DOUBLE LEG BRIDGE

1. Keep lying on your back.
2. Knees flexed, feet on the floor.
3. Arms straight by the side of your body.
4. Raise the pelvis from the ground towards the ceiling.
5. Hold for 10-15 seconds.
6. Repeat for 3-5 sets of 5-10 times.

The aim of this exercise is to strengthen the core muscles (dorsal and abdominal), as well as the thigh muscles (quadriceps and hamstrings). This is one of the final exercises someone has to do.

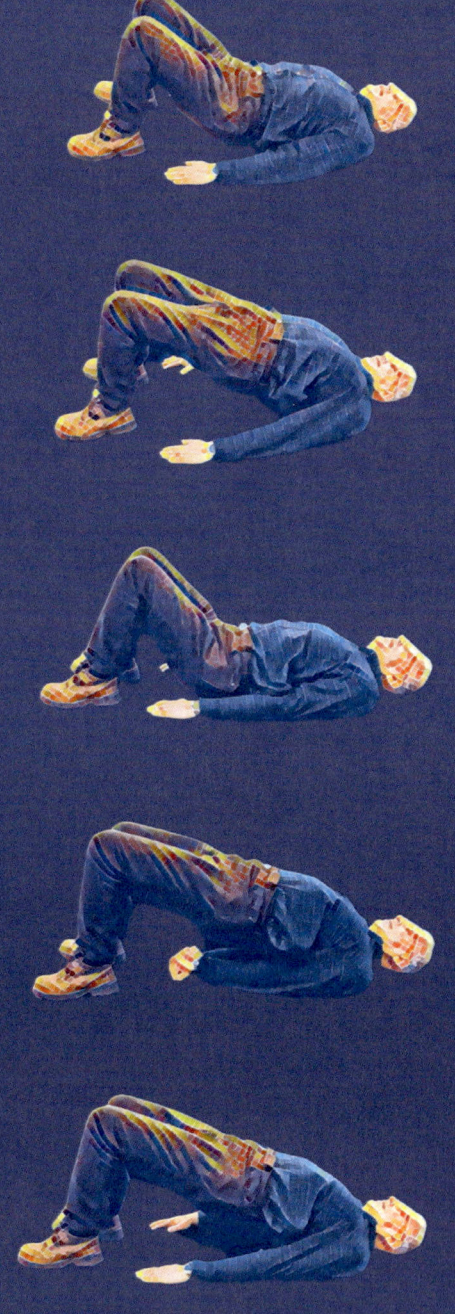

I. COW – CAMEL/CAT POSITION

COW

1. Get down on your hands and knees.
2. Relax your abdominal muscles and let your back "fall" towards the floor, creating a downward curvature.
3. Keep this extended position for 10 seconds.

CAT/CAMEL

1. Then, tighten your abdominal muscles and curve the back upwards like a hump.
2. Hold this position for another 10 seconds.
3. Repeat 3-5 sets 10-20 times.

The combination of these exercises creates contractions, as well as stretches to different muscle groups, depending on the position and the exercise being performed. The muscle groups involved are the abdominal and dorsal muscles, alternating between them.

Occasionally, it is possible for muscles to develop cramps. In such cases, please relax and reverse the movement.

COW

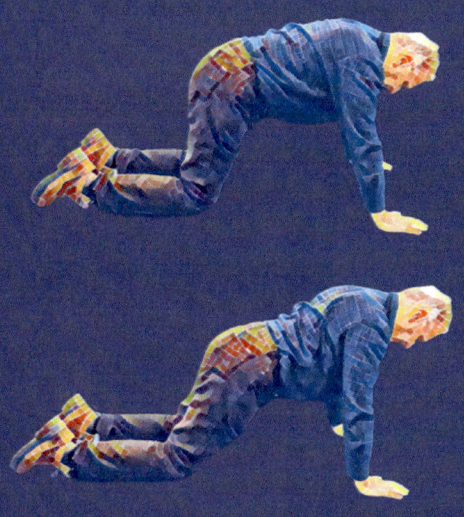

CAT/CAMEL

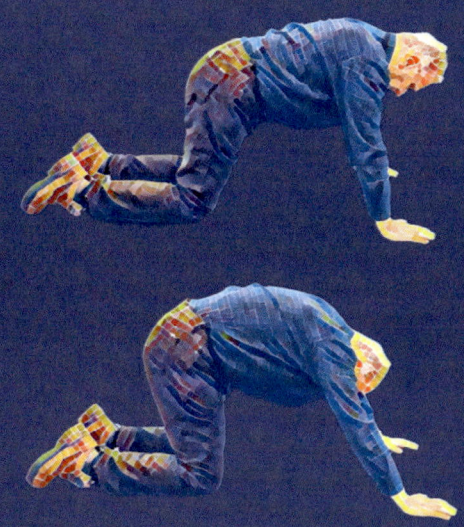

J. QUADRUPED – HALF SUPERMAN

1. Stay down on your hands and knees.
2. Lift one arm and extend it forward overhead.
3. Then lift the opposite leg and extend it straight backwards.
4. Hold this position for 5-10 seconds.
5. Repeat on the opposite side.
6. Do three sets of 10 repetitions.

During these exercises, there is a combination of isometric and isotonic muscle contractions involving several muscles. The main major muscles involved are the upper dorsal muscle known as the Trapezius, and the lower muscles known as the Glutei and Hamstrings.

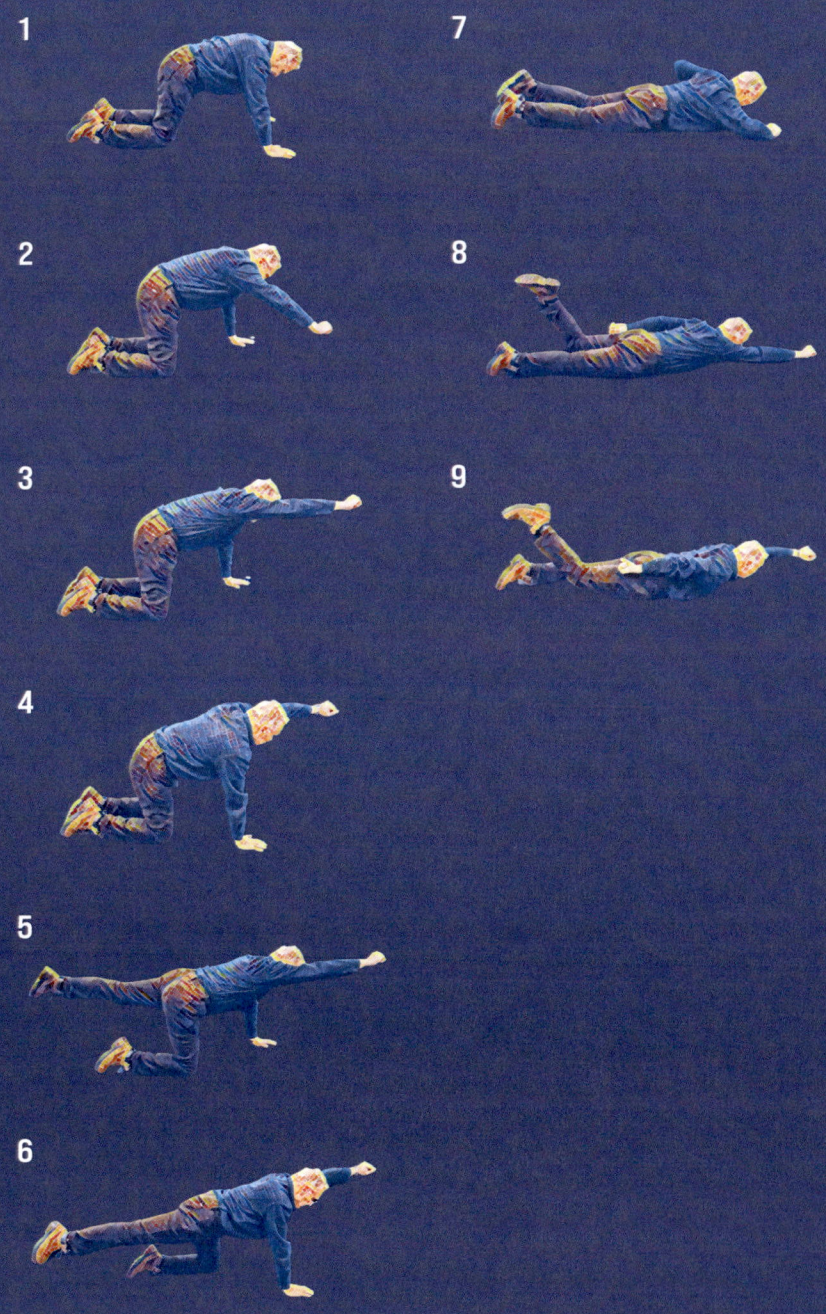

K. SUPERMAN

1. Lie on your stomach.
2. Extend both arms forward overhead.
3. Extend the leg straight backwards.
4. Tighten the muscles of your back in a way to lift part of your chest and your legs simultaneously off the floor.
5. Hold this position up to 10 seconds.
6. Repeat 3-5 sets, 10 repetitions.

This is a strengthening exercise.

Isotonic exercises involve a combination of different muscle groups, such as the dorsal muscles, the glutei and hamstrings.

IMPLEMENTATION 147

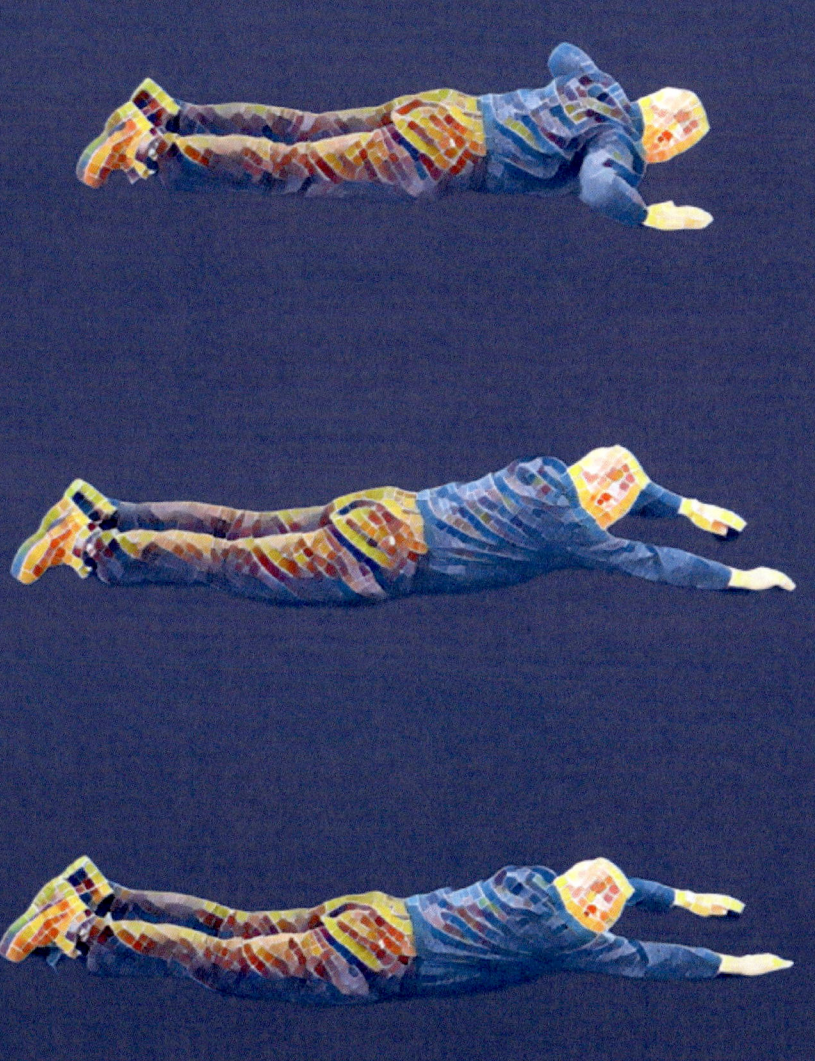

L. TURTLE

1. Stay down on your hands and knees.
2. Flex your hips and knees as your bottom moves towards your feet.
3. Extend your arms straight overhead with the palms on the ground.
4. Bring your face close to the floor.
5. Stretch your body as if you are reaching for something over your head, and at the same time, push your hips away from your shoulders.
6. Feel the stretching of the back muscles.
7. Hold this position for 10 breaths.
8. Repeat for 3 sets of 10 times.

This is a stretching exercise where you help the muscles to relax. Such an exercise could be at the end of any of the sessions.

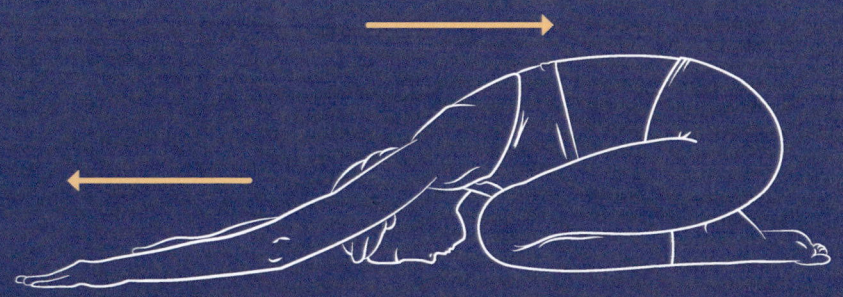
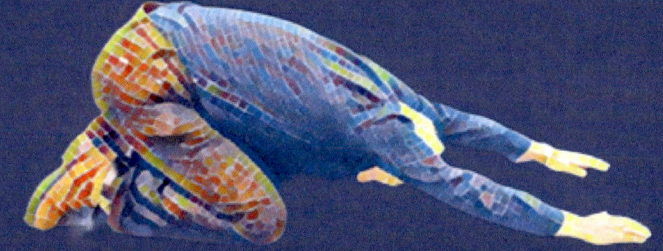

M. COBRA

1. Lie face down.
2. Place both hands at shoulder height.
3. Raise the upper torso from the ground as far as you can.
4. Keep the lower body relaxed.
5. Feel the squeeze of the dorsal muscles.
6. Stay in this position for 30 seconds or a minimum of 10 breaths.
7. Repeat 10 times.

HALF COBRA

- In case of difficulties with extending at the initial stages, stabilise the upper body on the elbows, instead of the hands.
- While in this position, keep the angle between the elbow and forearm at 90 degrees, with the forearm extended forward.

The back should be relaxed during these exercises, and the work should be done by the arms and shoulders.

The purpose of this exercise is to help gently shift a potentially anterior "displacement" of a mildly posteriorly bulging disc, as the anterior intervertebral space opens and allows the nucleus to be translated back into position.

Do not tense the muscles of the lower back at all.

COBRA

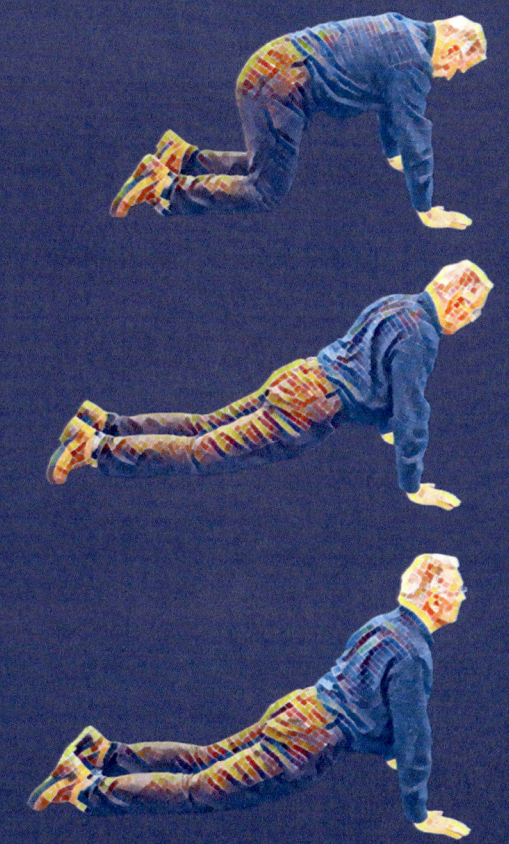

HALF COBRA

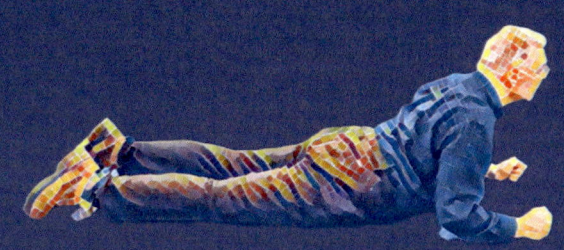

N. PLANK

1. Lie face down on the mat.
2. Place your elbows beneath your shoulders.
3. Extend your forearms on each side of your head.
4. Balance your upper body on your elbows, keeping the angle between your arm and forearm at 90 degrees.
5. Engage your back muscles and lift your pelvis off the floor.
6. Keep your legs straight and balance on your toes.
7. Hold this position for 30 seconds and repeat 5-10 times. Rest between repetitions.

Static isometric exercise for strengthening the abdominal and dorsal muscles, as well as the iliopsoas, quadriceps and glutei.

ALTERNATIVE PLANK

- If the described exercise is difficult to execute, instead of extending toes and balancing on toes, you can balance the lower part of your body on your knees.
- Progress to planking, when the dorsal muscles become stronger.

During these exercises, the dorsal muscles hold the pelvis in line while the combined anterior and lateral abdominals add their strength and assist the dorsal muscles. The iliopsoas assists the thigh muscles, which globally hold the position of the upper leg and lock the knee in extension. The calf muscles are also added to the equation to help stabilise the body. On the upper part of the body, the trapezius is one of the main muscles that play a role, assisted by the other dorsal muscles.

PLANK

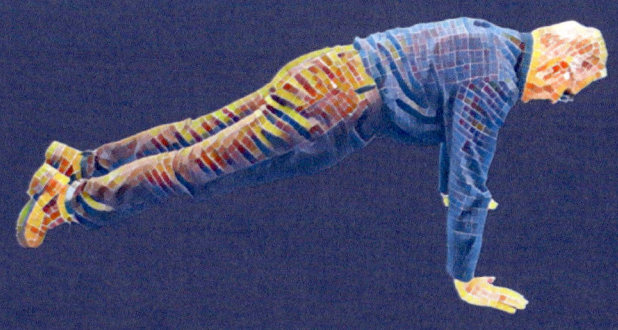

ALTERNATIVE PLANK

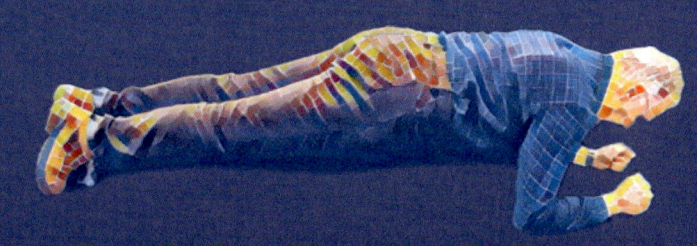

O. SIDE PLANK

1. Lie on your side with your legs, knees, and shoulders in a straight line.
2. Place your elbow under your shoulder and extend your forearm forward at a 90-degree angle.
3. Tighten your lateral abdominal muscles and lateral thigh muscles.
4. Raise your body (torso and pelvis) off the ground, balancing on your forearm-elbow complex on top and the lateral aspect of your foot at the bottom.
5. Hold this position for 30 seconds and repeat 5-10 times.
6. Take a rest between repetitions.
7. Repeat the exercise on the opposite side.
8.

ALTERNATIVE SIDE PLANK

Initially, if there is difficulty balancing the body on the elbow-forearm complex and feet, you can balance it on the elbow-forearm and the lateral aspect of the knee.

These are isometric exercises that mainly involve the lateral abdominal muscles, although other groups of muscles are involved as described in the previous pages.

Start with a duration of 10 breaths.

SIDE PLANK

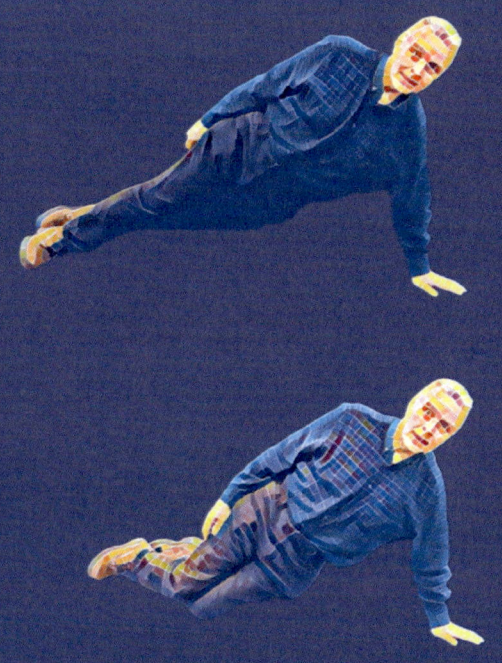

ALTERNATIVE SIDE PLANK

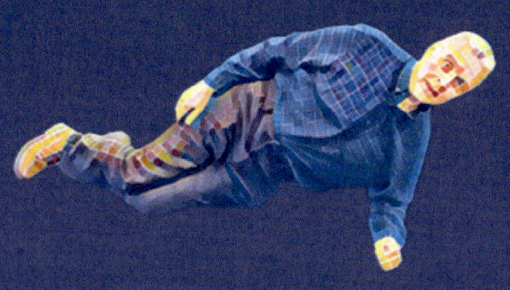

P. PRESS UPS

1. Lie face down on the mattress.
2. Place your hands under your shoulders.
3. Assume the Plank position – arms straight, body off the floor.
4. Bend your arms at the elbow joint.
5. Lower your body towards the floor.
6. Push your body up again.
7. Complete three sets of 10 repetitions.

Active isotonic strengthening exercises for the pectoral and upper arm muscles (triceps and biceps), but at the same time, isometric exercises for the abdominal and dorsal muscles.

ALTERNATIVE PRESS UPS

- Keep the Alternative plank position.
- Repeat the elbow movements as explained above.

ALTERNATIVE PRESS UP (VERSION 2)

- In case you have difficulty balancing with your hands extended on the floor, you can use other objects instead (such as a wooden box, side of the bed, or wall) and perform the same exercise.

These positions only help to reduce the load that goes through the upper body and facilitate you, in case of difficulties performing proper press-ups.

PRESS UPS

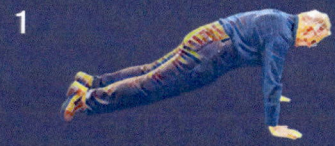
1

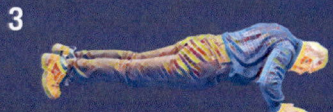
3

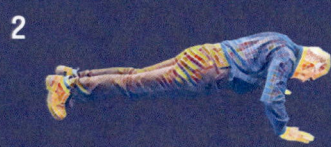
2

ALTERNATIVE PRESS UPS

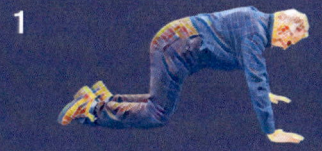
1

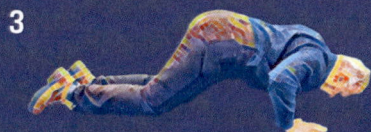
3

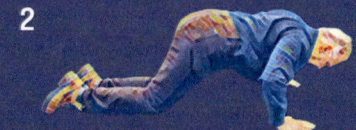
2

ALTERNATIVE PRESS UP (VERSION 2)

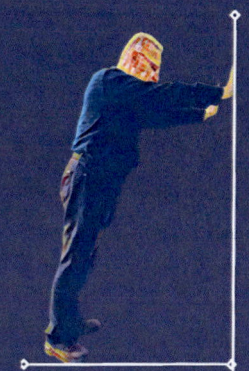
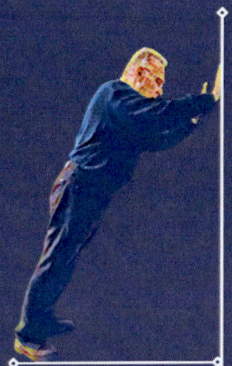
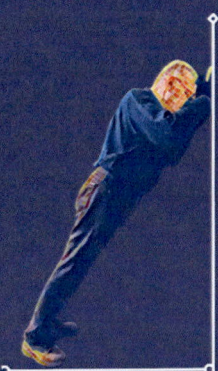

Q. ROTATIONAL STRETCHING OF BACK IN SITING POSITION

1. Stay in a sitting position, either on a chair or preferably on the floor. Keep one leg straight and bend the opposite leg, crossing it over the straight leg.
2. Twist your body from one side to the neutral position (neutral is when your face is looking forward).
3. The torso pivots over the extended arm that is placed on the floor behind you, in an attempt to stabilise yourself.
4. The other arm is placed across the knee of the bent leg, and the elbow touches the knee.
5. Push with your knee against the arm, forcing torso rotation.
6. During this exercise, you stretch the lower back as well as the external rotator muscles of the hip.
7. Repeat the same on the opposite side.
8. Do three sets with 15-20 repetitions for each set.

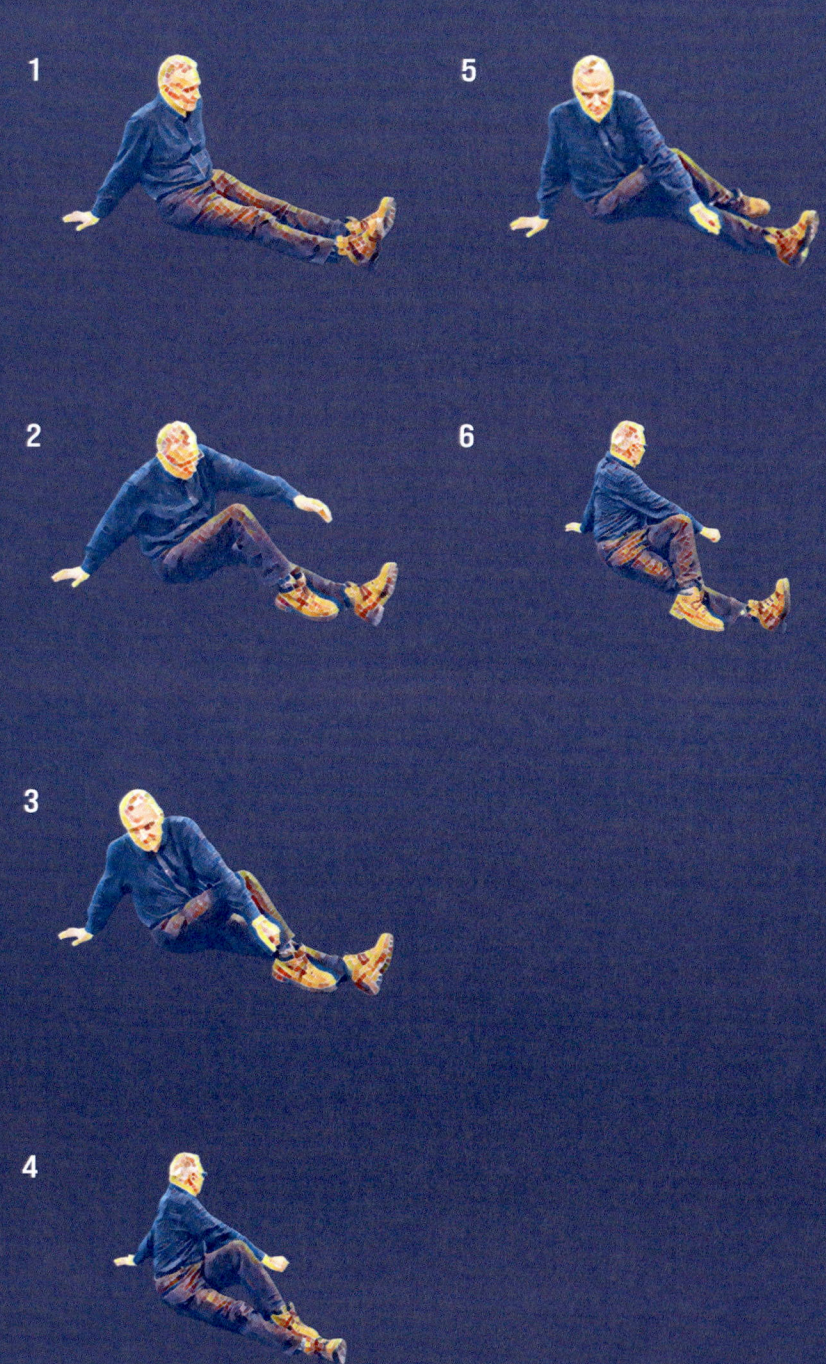

MUSIC – MOVIES

In this part, I will not elaborate much as everyone has their own favourite music. I like soft instrumental easy listening music as well as classical or even rock ballads. I am not telling you to change your musical taste because of the kind of music I am listening to. Listen to the music you like, although it has already been mentioned that music or movies play a significant role in hormonal secretion; hormones are responsible for our chronic pain improvement. Music has to "talk" to you. Personally, I load my music on my phone and when I have time, I listen to a part of it. This way, I am relaxing from a stressful day. The downtime was very beneficial to my depressed, anxious, and frustrated mind. I could read a book with some instrumental music playing in the background.

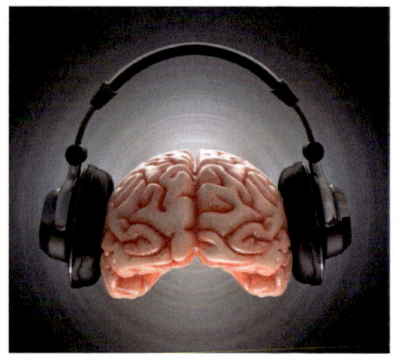

On top of that, I adjusted my taste in movies.

The books I was reading were inspirational books that were helping me change my habits and provide more information on the steps I needed to take to improve my situation. I really wanted to be free. Music is still my way of keeping to myself.

Spend a minimum of ten to fifteen minutes (10 – 15) per day, every day, listening to your favourite music, although there is even more improvement if the time spent increases to half an hour.

MEDITATION

I have a few options on this matter:
1. I would take long walks next to the ocean, on the beach, early in the morning, regardless of the weather conditions. Being close to the water and hearing the waves gives a great feeling of inner cleansing.

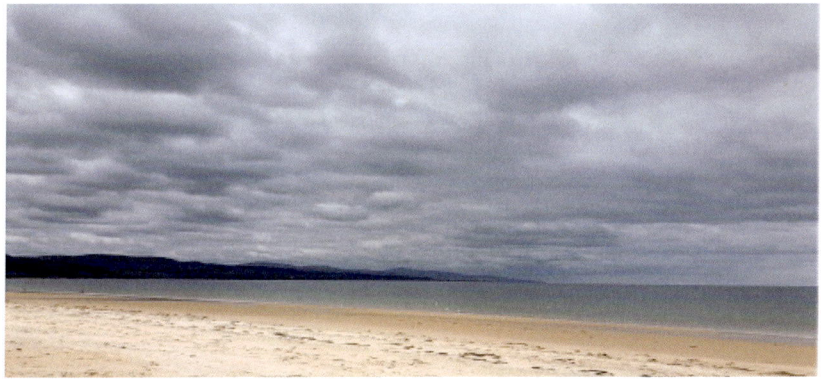

The sound of the waves and the rhythm of this sound were very comforting in my mind.

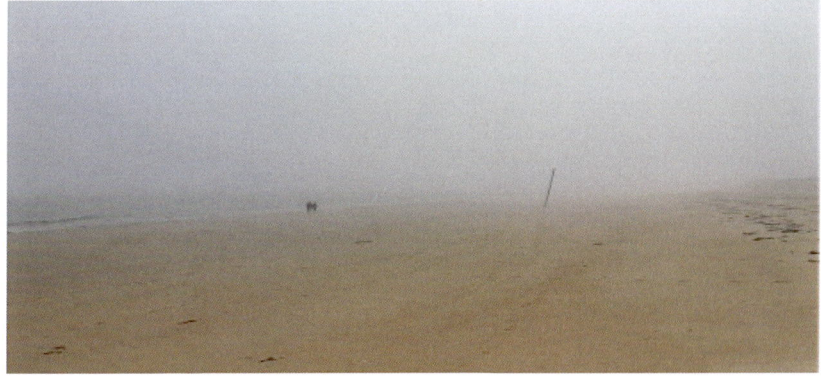

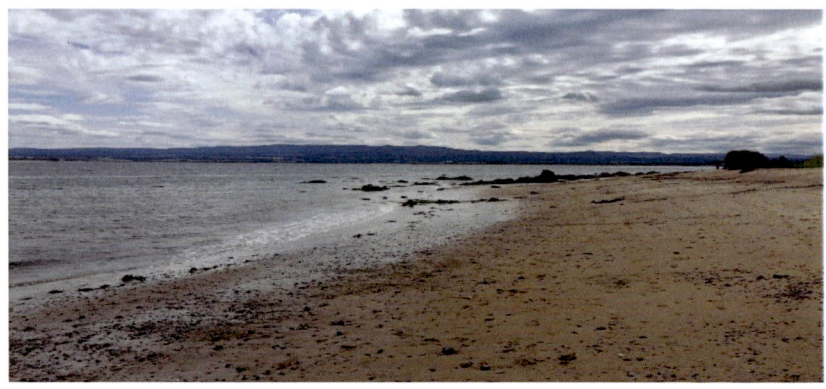

2. During my walks, I found this bench at the tip of the path on a small "cape." I spent hours sitting on it next to the sea at that small cape at the end of the round walking path, admiring the natural beauty. The connection with the water was great.

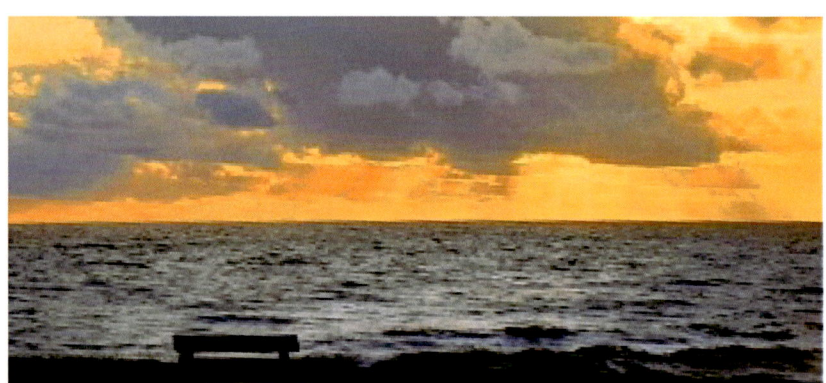

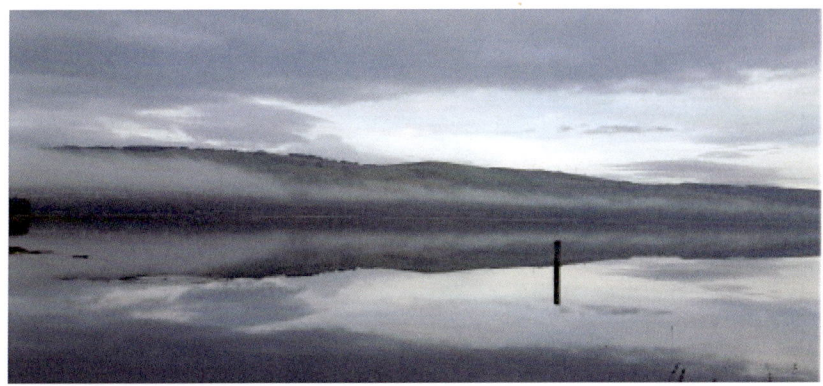

Nature has a great calming effect. Just seeing the reflection of the mist on the still water in the distance gives you a feeling of admiration. How does Nature really create this scenery? It is so calming.

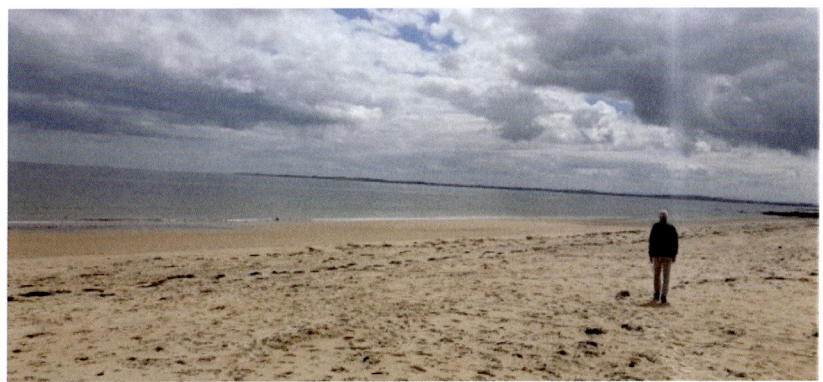

3. A walk through the forest, next to a river with waterfalls. The sound of the falling water is great, as it is the sound of nature calling you to be energised.

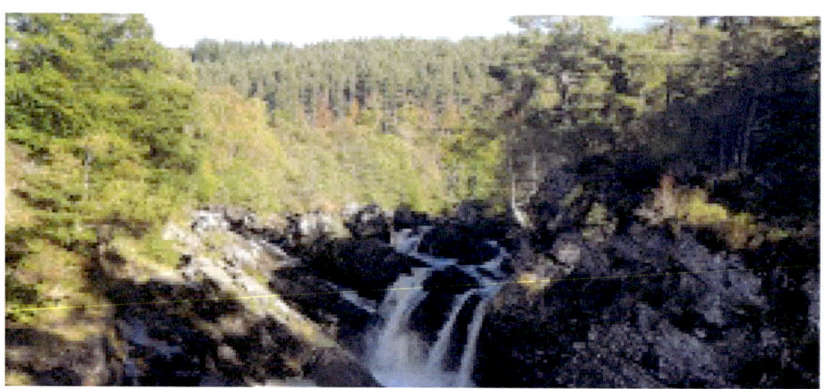

The flowing water takes away all the negative thoughts you have and carries them down to the sea.

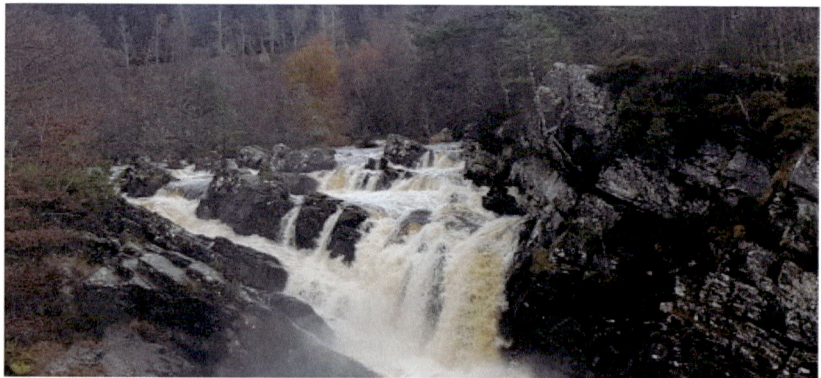

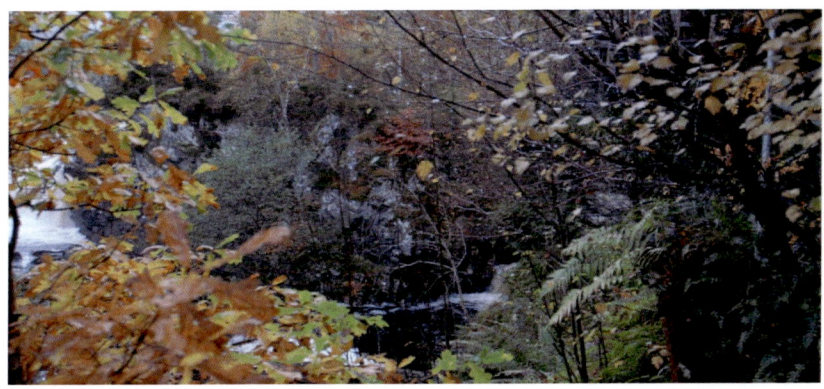

BREATHING EXERCISES

Under soft music, I was doing breathing exercises, concentrating within and finding pleasurable thoughts of my life.

This exercise is the only one that can be done outdoors or indoors and helps reduce stress and anxiety.

Sit in a comfortable seat, preferably with a straight back. Place both feet on the ground, and if you are at home, remove your shoes. Do not cross your legs. If possible, stay upright without touching the back of the chair. Close your eyes and feel the weight of your body. Focus on your breathing as you inhale and exhale. Breathe in through your nostrils and exhale through your mouth, following the journey of the air from your nostrils to your lungs and back out. Observe the movements of your chest and abdomen as you breathe. Pay attention to any pauses you take during your breathing. Control the duration of your inhalation and try to exhale for the same length of time. You can silently count 1, 2, 3 when you inhale and repeat the count when you exhale to achieve this.

As you do this exercise, your mind may lose concentration and start to wander. Do not panic; this often happens in the beginning. Gently guide your mind back to your breathing, just as you would guide a horse back on course while riding it. This way, you are controlling your mind and connecting it with the present moment. Soft music in the background may help if you are indoors.

During this breathing exercise, imagine that as the "dirty" air comes out of your lungs, you are also pushing out all unnecessary negative thoughts from your body. Visualise removing them from your inner self, just as you remove carbon dioxide.

Pay attention to any feelings you may have, such as anger, frustration, or anxiety. Acknowledge them and slowly think of a sunny place where you feel calm.

If you are outdoors and there is water nearby, let the sound of running water absorb into your mind, imagining that it is cleansing and carrying away all these negative emotions downstream, far away from you.

If you are indoors, imagine a light coming upon you. Let it travel through your head, down your spine, and into your feet, taking away all these heavy feelings to the core of the earth, where they are burned. Let this cleansing light fill your body with happiness and calmness.

When you are ready, bring your attention back to your breathing and slowly become aware of your surroundings. Open your eyes.

MENTAL AWARENESS

In this section we need to answer the following fundamental questions:
1. Where are you?
2. Where do you want to go?
3. Why do you need to do this?
4. What do you have to do to achieve change?
5. How will you do it?

WHERE ARE YOU?

This is the starting point. Accept your condition. You have back pain. You cannot deny it, but you can confront it. It all starts here. You need to answer honestly. Reflect deeply in your mind and confirm that this is point zero. You cannot achieve any goals if you don't know your present circumstances. Accept the realities of your life, let go of the judgmental view you have of yourself, and make the effort to begin the change. Be honest about your present situation. Remove any signs of self-pity and accept yourself as you are. If you don't know the starting point of your path at the beginning of your journey, you will not be able to map it.

How can you find it though? There are several reasons for you to be here in this moment. You either want to avoid pain or you have to find a happy result in your life, or maybe both. Possibly your back pain has not been treated to your satisfaction, either due to the proposed treatment itself or a lack of understanding about the condition. Perhaps you have not yet found a way to manage your back pain and find a compromise that allows you to live a more enjoyable life.

So stop and think about where you are now. What is your current situation? What are your physical symptoms? How do they influence your emotional well-being? How does your family or broader social environment react? What is your behaviour towards yourself or the people around you? What is your connection with a Higher Power? The most important question, however, is: what is your opinion about yourself?

Answer honestly, but also remember that you are still alive and blessed to be able to react and change your life for the better. Let these positive thoughts guide you and concentrate on them, but also analyse any negative feelings. You need to be aware of what you really need to replace with positivity. You need the energy to start and launch the beginning of your journey, like the fuel and energy necessary for the blast off of a rocket.t Cape Canaveral. The rocket consumes and burns tons of fuel to achieve a lift of starting the amazing journey. But all starts at Cape Canaveral. Find yours.

Write down your thoughts and feelings (mental and physical).

WHERE DO YOU WANT TO GO?

What is your destination? In six months or a year from now, what do you think you want to achieve? What kind of life do you want to have?

Possibly, this is the most difficult question someone could ask you to answer. The majority of people know the problems they have and can list them in detail, but they never analyse their destination. Perhaps they imagine a place without these specific problems. I use the word "analyse" because they are living with these day-to-day problems and have become accustomed to firefighting, forgetting that by creating a strategic plan, they may resolve the issues. This is the reason they don't think about their future goals. If someone has to resolve any issues, they need to know the end result and therefore, the end destination. You have to imagine your end result and create a path that you have to follow. Think of this destination as a lighthouse in the distance and try to get there. Be smart and avoid the rocks, though.

All of us remember the poster of the man who, by using his index finger, showed each of us and asked us to do something. During the Second World War, as we see in films, his words were "Your country needs you." Nowadays, he is asking us to donate blood or organs. But this shows the "Power of the Index Finger." We are following it.

Concentrate on positive thoughts and follow them. It is not easy or comfortable. You have to take uncomfortable action and go for it. If you want six pack muscles, photoshop one of your pictures where the six packs are evident and pin it on the fridge to see it every day. Same if you want to change your BMI. But on this picture, add some emotional thought. It is pointless to pin the picture and see it with an empty mind or think as you pass in front of the fridge, "I will be like this." You have to see the picture and vividly think "I will look like Hercules, strong and healthy, and to do this, I have to exercise because this is my goal."

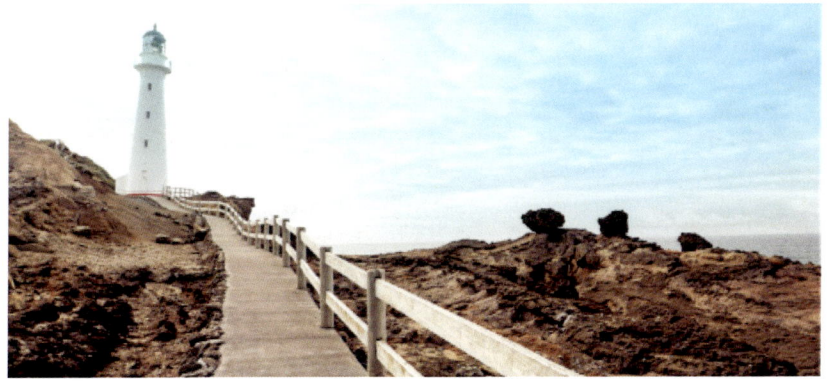

Focus on this future image, destination, or goal. Pretend that you are there, six or twelve months from now, and you are celebrating your achievement. During this party, someone comes up to you and asks you how you have done it. To answer this, you have to look back, follow the steps you walked from the start, and explain all this to that person. You know the steps. You have to be fluent. Describe all the way to your goal using colours and passion and be alive. Do not describe the story in black, grey, and white.

Now that you know the path, sit down and write what the goal you really want to achieve

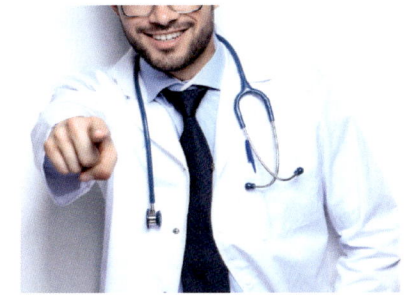

is, what will be your destination, and pretend you are there. Write down that you may want to live a life without pain or that you want six packs or that you have achieved a normal BMI, and now turn back and see the path you walked, all the steps taken, visualise every step, and write down how you achieved it.

Make a plan, a realistic plan. You have to achieve, but celebrate every single step of your achievement. This plan has to be down to earth. You will not be neither anxious nor depressed if you set unrealistic goals and you are unable to fulfil them. If your goal is to lose 20kg of weight in seven days, which is a fantasy, but you manage to lose 5kg, don't be unhappy. Your initial expectations were unrealistic, but celebrate the positive step you took towards your long-term goal, weight loss.

But all this, you have to write it vividly. Do not write the path, your plan, and your achievements in a bullet point list. Write it all with "colour."

For example, if you wanted more money, you will not write "I want money in the bank account" or "I want this expensive car," but you will imagine yourself within the car going to the beach and enjoying the sunshine with the rooftop down. This is the emotional picture. Create pictures. I hope it is clear.

On the other hand, as the plan is to manage the back pain, if you want to control your weight and visualise yourself with fewer kilos than before, elaborate on the picture. Write about your athletic, slim body. Write about the pleasure you will feel when you are in your swimsuit. Write about the speed you will have when you are running after your grandkids. Close your eyes and see the picture within your mind. Create an ideal movie of your future life. You need to add emotion. Emotion helps our imagination.

WHY DO YOU NEED TO DO THIS?

This is another question you have to think deeply about. Why do you want to change? Is it because you don't want to be in pain? Is this the only reason, or is it because the quality of your life is in ruins, and you want to make it better? Have you lost your job and you want to find a new one but cannot? Do you have problems with your partner, and are you upset about it? Is it because you have gained a lot of weight and want to lose it?

If any of the above is the reason, you have to find out the answers. But if you have a different goal, then find out the answer to a different question. As soon as you find that this is your purpose, you have to ask yourself if you have the energy to propel yourself toward this goal.

To answer all of this, you have to reflect within your soul and answer a series of questions. This may feel repetitive, but it is not entirely true. Grammatically, it is the same question, but the meaning of it is different every time, as it drives you deeper and deeper into your thoughts. Every question is based on the answer you give to the previous one. This was proposed and developed by my tutor and mentor, Dean Graziosi, who is an author, educator, founder of self-development, and a great believer in the change's education can achieve for all of us.

It is called the **7 Levels Deep** and the questions are:
1. What is important to you knowing what back pain is?
2. Why is important to you?
3. Why is important to you?
4. Why is important to you?
5. Why is important to you?
6. Why is important to you?
7. Why is important to you?

In every step, you have to ask "Why" based on the previous answer. This is what I mean when I say that the questions have a different meaning, even though they are grammatically the same.

Initially, I used a well-known tool for reflection called the De Bono Six Thinking Hats. The hats represent different perspectives: **White hat** for gathering facts, **Red hat** for analysing emotions, **Green hat** for focusing on creativity, possibilities, and new ideas, **Yellow** hat for exploring the positive aspects and symbolising optimism, **Black hat** for symbolising caution and critical thinking in analysing problems (do not overuse it), and **Blue hat** for focusing on how the situation is or should be managed. However, the 7 Levels Deep technique led me to a better understanding and created an emotional anchor for my reasoning.

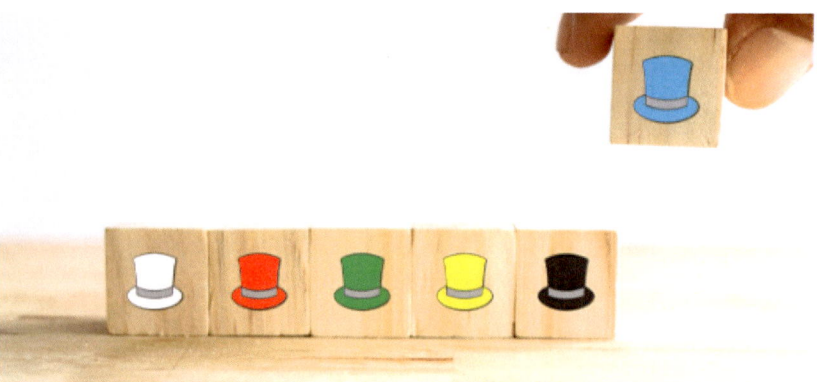

You need to find out why. By finding it, you will amplify your desire for the change you want. You have to write it down and engrave it in your brain. It is known that if you do this, you will find that the focal point is getting closer and bigger.

Let's use potential answers as examples to answer the 7 Level Deep questions:

1. What is important to you in knowing what causes back pain?
   I want to escape from the daily torture of pain and I want to understand what is causing it.
2. Why is it important to you to escape from the daily torture?
   I cannot live with the stiffness in my back every morning, and I want to feel relaxed and happy.
3. Why is it important to you to stop the stiffness and how would you feel relaxed?
   Every morning, it takes me a while to get out of bed and I need to take painkillers to improve my mobility. I am unsteady and have to rely on furniture for support until I can slowly improve my posture, and this creates a lot of anxiety. I don't know how long this will take, and it makes me unhappy.
4. Why is it important to you to become a happy person?
   Because these mood swings can affect my entire life. At work, I am moody and I fear that there may be a moment when I will speak in a different tone to one of the patients. I have lost my patience, and this is dangerous.
5. Why is it important to you to regain your patience?
   In order to serve people effectively, I need to have patience and listen to them and their problems and try to solve them. Without patience, I won't be able to serve anyone, and I will come across as an unpleasant person. I need to be able to control my emotions.
6. Why is it important to you to control your emotions?
   My emotions influence my behaviour, and this is affecting my family life. My spouse is becoming agitated because when she tries to help me, I have a fear that she will do something wrong, and I push her away. This makes me angry, angry at myself for my behaviour.

7. Why is it important to you to stop being angry?
Because this affects the well-being of my children, and they deserve to live in a calm, positive, and non-traumatic environment. This could create problems for their future, and I want to have a healthy, happy, safe, and confident family life.

While I may have answered some of your questions with these examples, please take a moment to honestly reflect and try to answer the 7 "why" questions in your own words.

WHAT DO YOU HAVE TO DO TO ACHIEVE CHANGE?

What are the tools or powers that you need to help you move forward and achieve your goals?

In my opinion, all of these tools are within your reach; you already possess them. You have your body, your own body, and your mind, your own mind. You are now capable of understanding how the body interacts with the mind and how you can utilise this knowledge and manipulate it in a way that allows you to achieve your goals. You need to take uncomfortable actions, change your beliefs, convince yourself that you can do it, and step out of your comfort zone to start taking action.

If you want a positive change in your situation, you must give up the attitude of defending your current circumstances. You need to be willing to change. Willingness is a state that empowers you to engage with your life and see situations from a new perspective.

"Where the willingness is great, the difficulties cannot be great"
— NICCOLO MACHIAVELLI

It requires focus, concentration, perseverance, determination, and certainty in yourself. If you change your beliefs and realise that all of us, including you, have enormous potential in our physical and mental reserves, you will be able to change the results to the level you desire if you take action. This action may be prolonged and will definitely take you out of your comfort zone and require a lot of work. It will not happen overnight.

Do not be afraid of failure. Embrace the paradox of seeing failure as a victory. There are two options in this argument. Failure is a victory because you subconsciously planned for it from the beginning. You may have never believed that your plan would be successful. It is similar to a failed marriage. You may have subconsciously thought that you do not deserve a successful relationship due to past experiences. So, you successfully "won" your failure as you had planned for it all along without knowing. On the other hand, failure can also be a victory because it represents a lesson that someone must learn from and not repeat. Considering all of this, you should not be afraid of failure, but at the same time, you must be positive and avoid failure by using the correct planned strategy.

You may wonder, are we certain about the future success of our actions?

Here we encounWter another paradox, the paradox of certainty. I would say that it is not possible to be certain of any success. If we do not venture beyond the surface of uncertainty and step out of our routine comfort zone, we will not improve our present circumstances, and this is certain. Chasing certainty is more or less chasing something that does not exist because nothing in life is certain except for the future demise of each one of us. So, if nothing is certain, we can say that everything is uncertain. Why then do we fear uncertainty when we live within it? It is the false feeling of comfort that numbs our mind. It is fear. So, stop fearing uncertainty and embrace it. Only then will you see change.

But you may argue that you have thoughts that everything will stay the same and nothing will change, and that everything will fail. These are negative thoughts. Do you have negative thoughts? Do not fear them. Everyone has them. They are part of our primitive brain. Do not let them define you. You are defined by your actions, not your thoughts. Those around you observe your actions, not your thoughts. Separate your thoughts from your actions. Act in a positive and assertive way, even if your brain fills with negativity. Negativity will continue to come to you if you allow it through inactivity. Fight back; persist in a routine that can push away any negative thoughts. Take positive action. This is the only solution. Action builds your confidence, and confidence helps you overcome any negativity. Be in control of yourself and your life. This is freedom.

> *"A man who cannot control self is not free"*
>
> — PYTHAGORAS

HOW WILL YOU DO IT?

What do you think you will need in order to achieve your goals?

Dr. Daniel Amen, renowned neuro-psychologist, has said in his teachings that you have to **love** your brain and support it. You have to provide it with the correct nutrition. Nutrition for the brain includes not only the correct substances that will reach it through the blood supply, but also the correct thoughts. He uses a nice terminology that creates a vivid picture. He states that you have to protect your brain from the ANTs (Autonomous Negative Thoughts), as these can harm your brain.

He emphasises that everyone needs to have positive thoughts and keep their brain happy.

Everyone knows what will make them unhappy. Try to reflect and find out the reasons for your unhappiness, write them down, and make it your goal to avoid them.

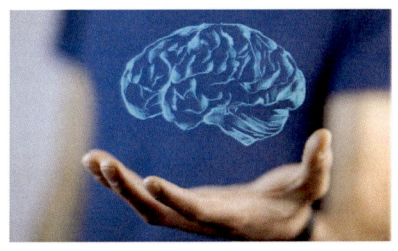

Let's see what I have done myself.

I already mentioned that I am a chronic low back pain sufferer for the last 25 years, and as such, I am in a position to fully understand how you are feeling and how pain is affecting your body function and mental well-being.

I sat down and wrote about all the unhappy moments and what created these feelings, whether mental or physical, and consciously started to avoid them. I can say that the physical ones were easier to detect, while the mental ones surfaced much later.

I used some tools available to overcome my anxiety and physical symptoms. I started reading and researching ways to improve my symptoms. I reminded myself about the anatomy of the region, as well as the way the spine works and the mechanics of the body. I spent hours going through different textbooks and research papers and reflected on and listed all the movements that were responsible for creating my symptoms. I used the tools I provided you in the motion and meditation section and focused on changing my appearance, as I had to change my BMI and improve my general health. I studied different books describing methods of diets and healthy food intake and committed to exercising.

In other words, I was trying to understand my body better. To achieve this, I had to change my mindset. I changed my habits, and in this way, I changed my life and now feel happier.

Reflecting on this part, I can easily tell you that by taking the uncomfortable action and transitioning from a sedentary life to an active one, I achieved the results I have now, and I am no longer in pain, except for occasional toothache-like discomfort that lasts only for minutes. However, I changed more than just the back pain. I improved my general health.

This is the reason why I believe that I can assist you by sharing my journey and experiences.

In this printed material, you have all the information that will help you understand how the spine functions and how you can improve your symptoms, and possibly everything you need to start your journey towards a better life without pain. You need to find the ways that work for you and implement them, so that you can realise your change. Please, I urge you to take action upon it.

MARKING DOWN

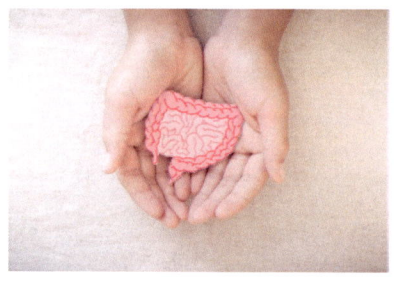

As mentioned in my previous exercise, I lost weight, but my BMI was still not correct. To improve this, I bought books that explain different ways of losing weight. I followed some of the described methods, but I was unable to achieve my desired result. I experimented with several healthy diets until I found one that made me happy. I started losing weight while also feeling satisfied. I replaced many of my meals with vegetables and salads. At the same time, I made sure to consume the right amount of protein by adding either fish or lean poultry to my diet. Red meat was very rarely included, but not completely eliminated from my diet. I completely eliminated sodas, and alcohol, only red wine, as well as salt and sweets were consumed very rarely. I also had to take care of my gut.

In addition, intermittent fasting was added, if you wish to. The first ten (10) days of fasting were very difficult. My strategy to cope with this was to keep myself busy, trying to avoid giving in to my cravings. Further experimentation was done to see what could work better. Initially, a 16:8 fasting schedule was followed (16 hours of fasting and 8 hours to eat. Be careful; do not overeat during the 8 hours you are allowed to eat. It is not helpful at all). Following this, I switched to a 2:5 schedule and I can say that it is working better for me as I am complementing this with my exercise regimen.

It is evident that I have implemented intermittent fasting and increased my intake of lean meat, fiber, and reduced carbohydrates and fats, except for olive oil.

I have brought back the wise words of the father of Medicine.

Hippocrates stated *"Let food be the medicine and medicine be the food."*

This is true. You need to follow the rules and have a balanced intake of a variety of nutritious foods that will benefit your body.

Additionally, keep your microbiome happy and your body rejuvenated by practicing autophagy.

But really, if you ask me, I don't think that only the diet itself makes the difference. It was my discipline to count my calories and ensure that I did not exceed the calculated amount for me.

I downloaded an app on my phone and started inputting everything I ate into it. The app automatically calculated my calories. I recorded everything and did not cheat. This is the reason I managed to control my weight.

Remember that BMI control is a journey in itself, based on the physical and mental changes your body goes through. To reverse these changes, you need to transform yourself physically and mentally, and be prepared to accept that traveling from A to Z may be difficult in one continuous journey. You may need to accept that stopping at K for a while is beneficial, and re-planning may be necessary.

You need to undergo transformation. To achieve this, you need to believe in yourself and make changes. You need to have integrity, meaning that you will follow and make your plan a reality within the timeframe you set. This is directly linked to self-respect and self-discipline. To reach your goal, you need to plan to take small achievable steps, which will boost your confidence. Being confident will enhance your ability to change your beliefs as you see the difference realistically. Do not lose faith in case of delays along your journey, and if you have someone nearby who can assist you in your journey, don't hesitate to seek their help. Humans are social animals. A friend will support you and help you on your journey, highlighting your achievements and not your failures. Stay positive.

In summary, the elements you need to complete your journey are integrity, dignity, discipline, attention to detail, perseverance, focus, inner light, patience, becoming part of a positive and helpful community, and above all, honesty. Be honest with yourself and others. Have your values and act according to them.

> FINALLY, I AM NOT GOING TO SUGGEST ANY OF THESE SCHEMES OF EITHER DIET OR FASTING PATTERNS, DIRECTLY TO YOU, AS WHAT WORKED WITH ME MAY NOT WORK WITH YOU. THIS IS MY JOURNEY, AND MY PURPOSE IS TO SHARE WITH MY EXPERIENCES WITH YOU. THIS IS MATERIAL IS FOR EDUCATIONAL PURPOSES. PLEASE KEEP WHAT YOU THINK IS RELEVANT TO YOU.
>
> BASE YOURSELF ON YOUR OWN CULTURAL AND INTELLECTUAL BACKGROUND AND ACCEPT WHAT MATERIAL MATCHES WITH THIS. FIND WHAT WORKS FOR YOU THROUGH EXPERIMENTATION AND ASK YOUR PERSONAL PHYSICIAN FOR ANY FURTHER ADVICE.

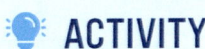
ACTIVITY

Write down what you need to avoid and make it a goal to eliminate them from your life.

Choose the exercises you are able to do.

Find ways to meditate.

Design your diet with or without the help of a physician but stay dedicated to the instructions and measure everything.

Answer your five M and seven level deep questions repeatedly.

EPILOGUE

Let's go back and discuss my response to the statements made by my female patient, the woman who wanted to go to Switzerland.

I offered to go with her on the journey, trying to make her understand the necessity of finding a solution to her problems and the reasons why we must stay alive.

We discussed the motion and exercises she had to perform. I helped her understand the benefits of exercising in water and the strain it would spare her osteoporotic bones, as well as how it could increase her mobility.

When she recognised this, we moved on to music. She liked all the soft music from the 50's, especially Paul Anka. I asked her if she used to dance in the past and her face lit up. I knew about a local club where people her age gathered almost daily, and they had dancing competitions once or twice a week. I promised her that I could find a driver through social services who could pick her up once a week and take her to the club. There, she could listen to her favourite music and possibly try dancing for 3-4 minutes, if she wanted.

I asked her to download an app on her phone for her music and play it when she wanted to relax at home. She could close her eyes and immerse herself in the melodies. This could help relax her muscles and react less to any discomfort.

Then we discussed mental awareness. I explained that her degenerative spine could not be changed, but her osteoporosis could improve with the right diet, medications, and movement. We discussed the course of action, and her attitude changed. The idea of potential improvement made her happier, and the smile returned to her face.

Finally, we discussed her diet and the medications she needed to take.

At the end of the consultation, she got up from the chair. Despite her awkward movements, her smile never left her face. She shook my hand firmly and left happy.

We had found the reason why she needed to follow this course of action, what she needed to do, and how she needed to do it.

I saw her about 4 months later. She was dressed more elegantly than before. She told me that her symptoms had improved, and she was happy and full of enthusiasm as she found out that her daughter-in-law was pregnant. She was looking forward to seeing and taking care of her grandchild. She never mentioned Switzerland again. If you ask whether her spine changed, the answer is no, she had the exact same spine. The only thing that changed after she learned how the spine works was her plan of action towards her spinal problems. She started to move, found ways to relax her mind, and because of that, her body changed. She changed her views about her life, and the new grandchild was a gift from heaven for her, giving her a purpose to live a longer and happier life.

For all of us, please apply the Epicurean Tetrapharmakos (four-part cure) and especially the fourth part of it: "What is terrible is easy to endure." Epicurus, the Greek philosopher, believed that "Continuous pain does not last long, even if it is extreme. It will only be present for a short period, and we have the ability to overcome it if we can recognise our physical and mental limits, and become confident that pleasure will follow the pain and nothing else."

Finally, here are two pictures from some research to serve as reminders and help you understand that simple activities can help you, and that emotions are something that affect the whole body.

HAPPINESS CHEMICALS AND HOW TO HACK THEM

DOPAMINE (THE REWARD)
- Complete a task
- Do self-care activities
- Eat food
- Celebrate little wins

SEROTONIN (THE MOOD STABILIZER)
- Meditate
- Run
- Expose under the sun
- Walk in nature
- Swim
- Cycle

OXYTOCIN (THE LOVE HORMONE)
- Play with a pet
- Play with a baby
- Hold hands
- Hug family
- Give compliment

ENDORPHINS (THE PAIN RELIEF)
- Laugh
- Use essential oils
- Watch comedy
- Eat dark chocolate
- Exercise

💡 ACTIVITY

Reflect and write down a journal of all thoughts applying to the 5 P's, 5 M's, and do the 7 Level Deep.

Reflect and find the reasons why your back pain is getting worse.

Become aware of your habits and daily thoughts that are linked to your back pain. Eliminate the negative thoughts and replace them with positive actions.

Plan your ideal future and work towards it; one step at a time.

Apply the exercises and increase your movement.

Move away from your sofa.

Plan the first task you need to do and concentrate on it. Once you are satisfied and focused, plan the next task to give attention to. Do not get obsessed with only one goal. Assess your ability to achieve the goals separately, taking one step at a time so you can plan the steps to reach your final goal.

Change your attitude towards mechanical low back pain; initially, it is your friend and if you perceive it as an enemy, try to go back to having a friendly relationship with it. Do not fight it, but "negotiate" with it.

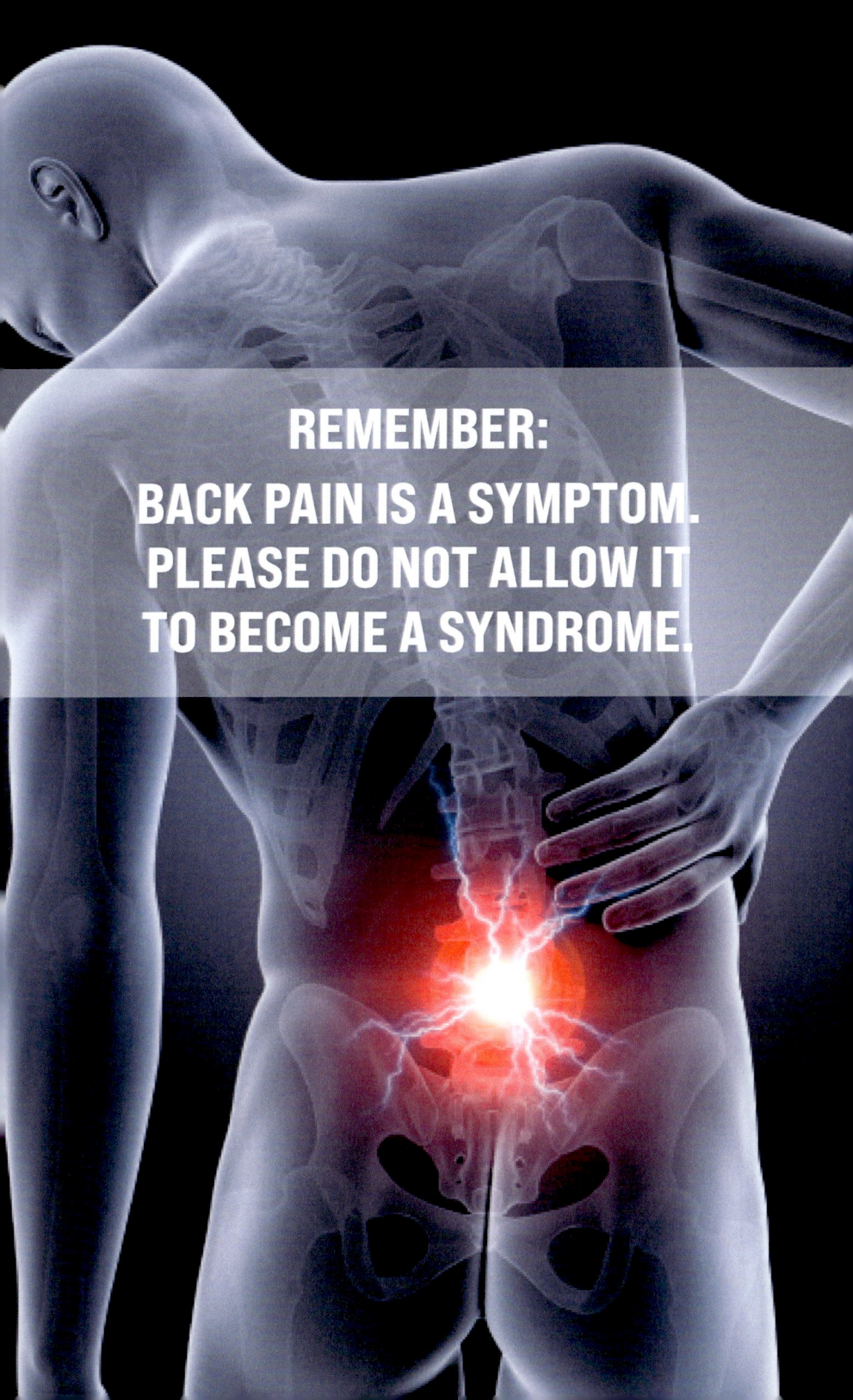

ONCE AGAIN, I AM REMINDING YOU THAT THIS IS ONLY AN EDUCATIONAL GUIDE FOR MANAGING SPECIFIC LOW BACK PAIN SYMPTOMS AND IT IS NOT A SUBSTITUTE FOR A MEDICAL CONSULTATION. YOU MAY TAKE FROM IT WHAT IS RELEVANT TO YOU ACCORDING TO YOUR CULTURAL AND INTELLECTUAL BELIEFS AND DISCARD THE REST.

IMPORTANT NOTICES / DISCLAIMERS

The depicted experience may not be considered as typical. Your background, education, experience, and work ethic may differ. This is used as an example and not a guarantee of success. Individuals do not track the typicality of their students' experiences. Your results may vary.

The contents of this training, such as text, graphics, images, and other material, are intended for informational and educational purposes and not for the purpose of providing medical or mental health advice. The contents of this training are not intended to substitute for professional medical advice, diagnosis, and/or treatment. Please consult your medical professional before making changes to your diet, exercise routine, medical regimen, lifestyle, and/or mental health care.

This is not a medical consultation or medical advice. It is a guide to be followed, aiming to improve the quality of your life. You can keep all necessary material and discard what is not working for you.

The stories shared during the sessions of the modules are true experiences of mine personally or of patients who crossed paths with me during consultations many years ago. No personal details are shared within the course that could make them identifiable to anybody.

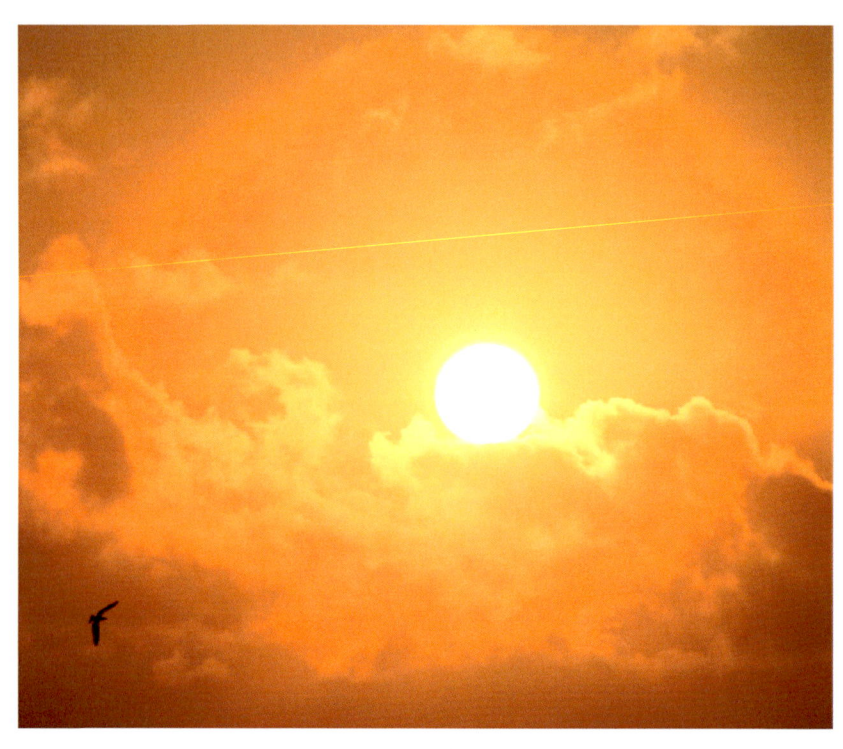

Follow the Light

EVALUATION

I would be grateful if you could take the time to complete the following questionnaire and email it to faceyourbackpain1@gmail.com:

1. Please indicate the appropriate grading on the following table (1 being the least relevant and 5 being the most relevant to you).

STATEMENTS	1	2	3	4	5
Was the content something you were expecting?					
Was the given information easy to understand?					
Were the illustrations clear?					
Did this material improve your knowledge?					
Was the material useful to you?					
Do you feel better after this?					

2. Please write below your opinion on what we can do better.

3. Please answer the following questions:
    - What were you like before the course?
    - How did the course made you feel?
    - What did you like most about it?
    - What changes have you made, following the course?

Thank you very much for allowing
me to share my experience
with you and serve you.

Thank you

www.ingramcontent.com/pod-product-compliance
Lightning Source LLC
Chambersburg PA
CBRC100215040426
42333CB00035B/70